AF712028

Cancer

Norra Tannenhaus

American Family Health Institute™

Medical Board

Stanley J. Dudrick, MD
Clinical Professor of Surgery
University of Texas Medical School, Houston, Texas

Jo Eland, RN, PhD
Assistant Professor, University of Iowa
Iowa City, Iowa

Dennis E. Leavelle, MD
Consulting Pathologist, Department of Laboratory Medicine
Mayo Clinic, Rochester, Minnesota

Julena Lind, MN, RN
Director of Education, Center for Health Information, Education and Research
at California Medical Center, Los Angeles, California

Ara G. Paul, PhD
Dean, College of Pharmacy, University of Michigan
Ann Arbor, Michigan

Richard Payne, MD
Clinical Assistant Neurologist, Memorial Sloan-Kettering Cancer Center
New York, New York

William R. Truscott, MD
Diplomate, American Academy of Family Practice, Lansdale Medical Group
Lansdale, Pennsylvania

SPRINGHOUSE CORPORATION
SPRINGHOUSE, PA.

Program Director
Stanley Loeb

Clinical Director
Barbara McVan, RN

Art Director
John Hubbard

Editors
Jay Hyams
Susan Cass

Editorial Services Supervisor
David Moreau

Production Manager
Wilbur Davidson

The charter of the American Family Health Institute is to research and produce high-quality publications that enhance the health of individuals and their families. Essential to health are physical, emotional, and social well-being, not just the absence of illness or infirmity. The Institute's Medical Board has produced the *Health and Fitness* books to share up-to-date and authoritative information that can give readers greater personal control over their health maintenance.

© 1986 by Springhouse Corporation, 1111 Bethlehem Pike, Springhouse, Pa. 19477

All rights reserved. Reproduction in whole or part by any means whatsoever without written permission of the publisher is prohibited by law. Printed in the United States of America.

Library of Congress Cataloging-in-Publication Data
Tannenhaus, Norra, 1953-
Cancer.
(Health and fitness series)
Includes index.
1. Cancer—Popular works. I. Brunner, Lillian Sholtis. II. American Family Health Institute. Medical Board. III. Title. IV. Series.
[DNLM: 1. Neoplasms—popular works. QZ 201 T167c]
RC263.T345 1986 616.99'4 85-30263
ISBN 0-87434-026-8

The procedures and explanations given in this publication are based on research and consultation with medical and nursing authorities. To the best of our knowledge, these procedures and explanations reflect currently accepted medical practice; nevertheless, they can't be considered absolute and universal recommendations. For individual application, treatment suggestions must be considered in light of the individual's health, subject to a doctor's specific recommendations. The authors and the publisher disclaim responsibility for any adverse effects resulting directly or indirectly from the suggested procedures, from any undetected errors, or from the reader's misunderstanding of the text.

Contents

Cancer

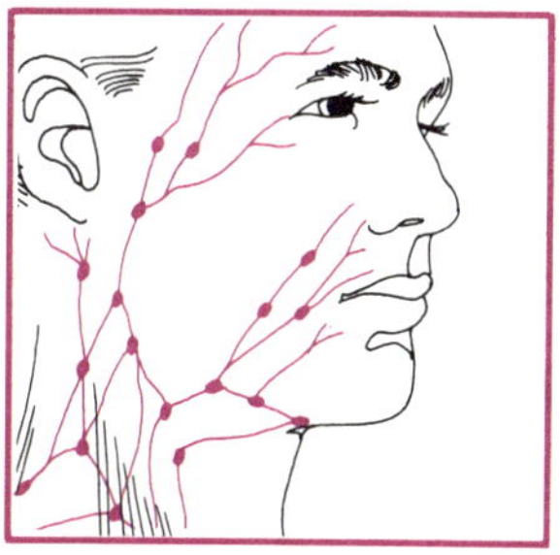

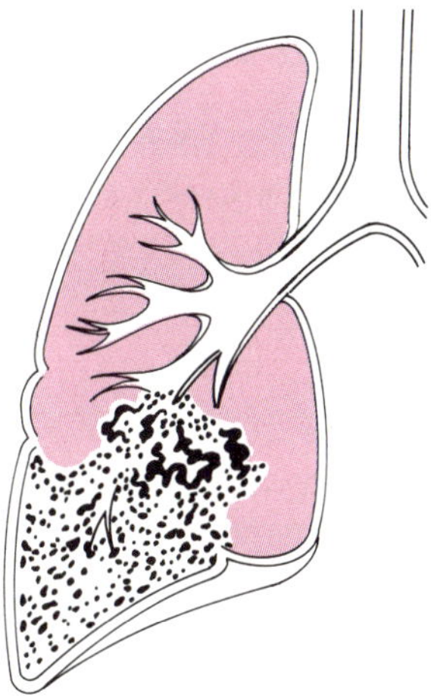

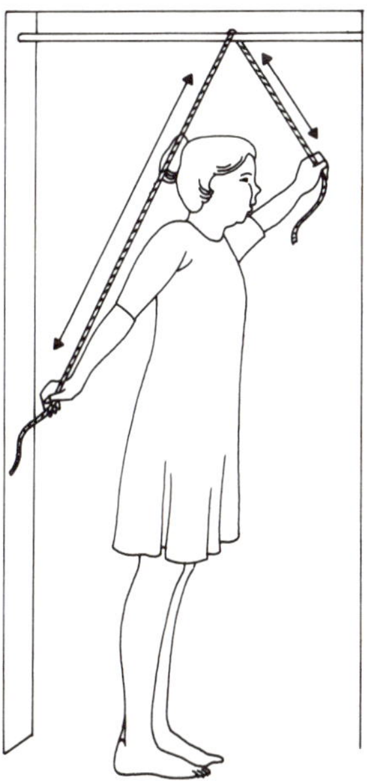

1 Knowing the enemy

Avoiding the risk of cancer

The cancer death rates would drop even more if people avoided some obvious risk factors. The first, of course, is smoking. The relationship between smoking and lung cancer is no longer in doubt. Following certain dietary guidelines could also reduce the risk of developing cancer:

- *Avoid eating fats.*
- *Eat more fruits, vegetables, and whole grain cereals.*
- *Eat salt-cured, smoked, and charcoal-broiled foods only in moderation.*
- *Drink alcoholic beverages only in moderation.*

For more on diet and cancer, see pages 18 to 23.

Americans fear cancer more than any other disease. Some people equate a cancer diagnosis with a death sentence, while others view it as being condemned to a lifetime of pain, disability, and disfigurement. The high occurrence of cancer today can even be seen as an indictment of modern life: certain cancers occur most frequently in people who smoke, drink alcoholic beverages, and eat rich foods. And cancer is partly mysterious: we still don't know exactly what triggers it or exactly how to treat it.

Some cancer statistics are indeed grim. Experts estimate that 1 out of every 4 people will develop cancer —that's about 54 million people in this country. According to the American Cancer Society, cancer struck more than 900,000 people in 1985 and killed more than 450,000. Cancer kills more children between the ages of 3 and 14 than any other disease.

But there's another side to this story. Three million people alive today fought cancer and won. Death rates from the major forms of cancer either have declined or leveled off in the past 50 years. The one exception is lung cancer, the death rates from which continue to soar.

This general decline in death rates has been most marked in children, reflecting the great strides doctors have made in treating and curing the childhood cancers. Fifty years ago, fewer than 1 in 5 cancer patients—about 20 percent—were alive 5 or more years after treatment. Today, about 3 out of 8 patients, or 39 percent of the people who got cancer in 1985, will be alive in 1990. These numbers could be even better. The American Cancer Society estimates that 160,000 cancer deaths could have been prevented had those people gone in sooner for diagnosis and treatment.

Cancer is a highly complex disease. It occurs in almost every kind of creature: animals, fish, and even plants. In humans, it's been known since ancient times. We talk about cancer as though it were a single disease, but it's actually more than 100 different diseases. Each kind behaves in a different way. Oat cell lung cancer, for example, is vastly different in symptoms and prognosis from a malignant melanoma. Cancers differ in their ability to spread, the predictability of their behavior, and their response to different kinds of treatment. Because of this, people naturally view cancer with confusion. To get the full perspective on cancer, you have to know what it is, how it develops, and how it spreads.

Common cancer warning signs

- *Weight loss without a diet*
- *Sores that don't heal*
- *Indigestion that persists*
- *Difficulty in swallowing*
- *Swollen glands in the neck or armpit*
- *Lump in breast*
- *Change in cough*
- *Change in bowel habits*
- *Change in urination habits*
- *Unusual bleeding*
- *Blood in urine or stool*
- *Changes in color or size of a wart*
- *Changes in vision*

What cancer is

Healthy cells normally reproduce by dividing: one cell into two, the two into four, the four into eight, and so on. Every cell has strict, inherited limits on how large it can grow and how many times it can reproduce. That's why, for example, humans are bigger than houseflies and smaller than whales. The primary characteristic of cancer cells is that they bypass these limits on growth—they reproduce uncontrollably, forming a lump called a tumor. By doing so they destroy the normal tissue around them and take nutrients from healthy cells. They also release enzymes that allow them to invade other organs. As a cancer grows, it may shed cells into the blood or lymph, which can carry them to more distant organs, where they may settle and begin growing again. These distant settlements are called metastases. Once a cancer has metastasized, or spread, the chances of curing it decrease greatly. That's why early detection of cancer is so important.

Normal lung

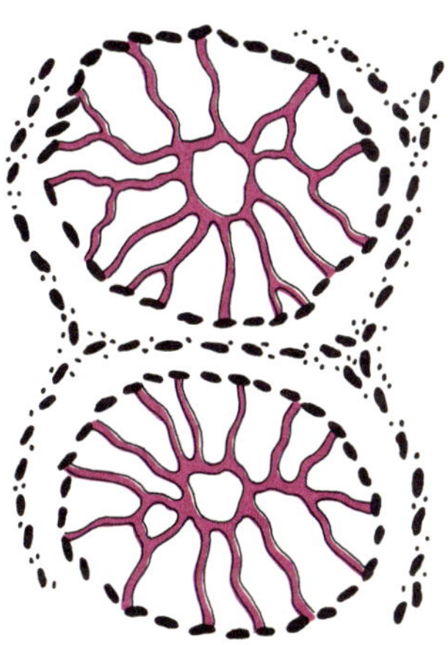

Healthy cells are thin, orderly in arrangement, and fairly uniform in size and shape. Those above surround glands in the colon.

Cancerous lung

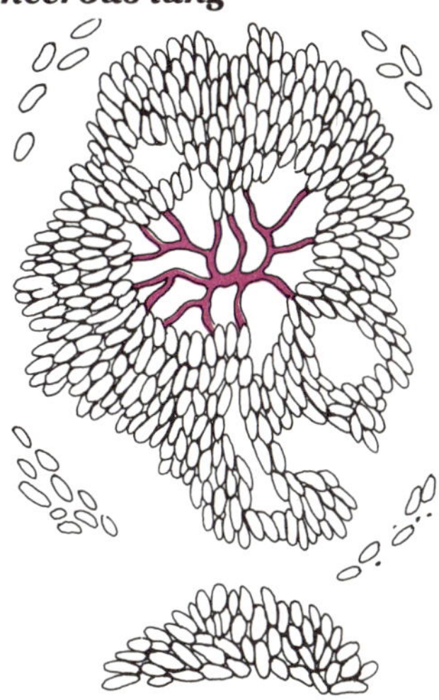

Cancer cells are thick, disorderly in arrangement, and various in size and shape. Those above have invaded a gland in the colon.

The birth of a cancer cell

Cancer cells arise from normal cells in the body. To understand how they do this, you'll need to know a little about a cell's genetic structure.

Each cell's genetic information is encoded in a substance called deoxyribonucleic acid, or DNA. When a cell reproduces, its DNA reproduces along with it, so the same genetic material is carried from one cell to another. The DNA contains messages for every trait in a cell in units called genes. For example, one set of genes may direct a certain cell to produce insulin (a

How a carcinogen causes a mutation in DNA

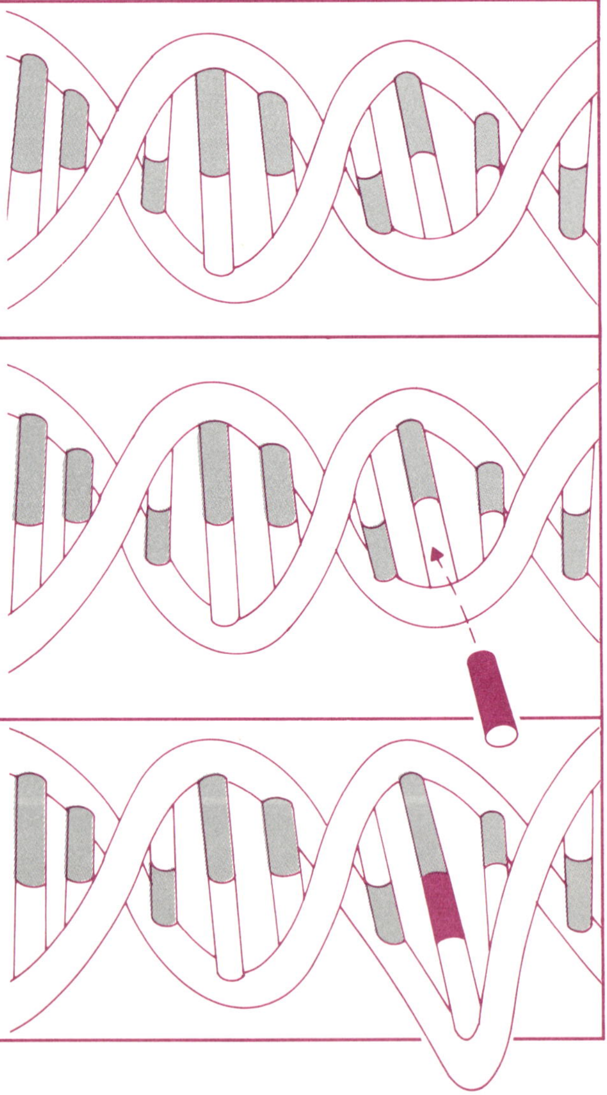

Normal DNA

Bound DNA
A carcinogen such as benzopyrene with components found in cigarette smoke can bind DNA, leading to a distortion.

Distorted DNA
A distortion in the DNA results.

hormone important for regulating sugar in the body), while a different set of genes may tell another cell to transmit nerve impulses. A change, or mutation, in a cell's DNA may have drastic consequences, since it can lead to the transmission of a faulty message. In the most extreme cases, mutations can cause deformity or even death.

Carcinogens—cancer-causing substances—probably cause a mutation in a cell's DNA. The result of this mutation maybe a malignant tumor, although it may be years before a tumor actually develops. Scientists now believe that carcinogenesis is a two-step process. Step one is called initiation; step two, promotion.

During initiation, an irreversible change occurs in a cell's genetic message. When an initiated cell divides, the new cell also carries the altered message, which is then passed on to subsequent generations of cells. If no further damage is done, the cells may continue to function normally, and no problem may ever be detected. For a cell to become cancerous, promotion must occur. One of the mysteries still facing scientists is how promotion enlarges on the effects of initiation, but promotion can occur months after initiation and still lead to cancer. It does this by speeding up the cells' reproduction rate and changing their character at maturity. The process must always happen in the right sequence: initiation first, and then promotion. Exposure to promotion without initiation won't cause cancer.

Some substances function as initiators, others act as promoters, and some, the complete carcinogens, act as both. Many environmental substances thought to cause cancer may not be complete carcinogens but, rather, initiators or promoters. Some chemicals may serve both functions, depending on the dose you're exposed to. For example, saccharin is thought to be a strong promoter, a weak initiator, and a weak carcinogen. Cigarette tars are both initiators and promoters. A high-fat diet, linked to colon cancer, may stimulate the production of hormones that act as promoters upon cells that have already been initiated by something else.

Another factor is at work. Our bodies come equipped with a regulated immune system that detects and destroys invaders. Many experts believe that cancer cells arise all the time, but the immune system finds and kills them. Then, one cell may arise that is capable of avoiding detection, and it gives birth to

Types of cancer

One-third of all malignant lung tumors are oat cell carcinomas. These are small, tightly packed, round or oval or spindle-shaped cells that usually spread along the tubes of the lymphatic system, rather than form large, bulky masses.

Malignant melanomas are the most serious kind of skin cancers. Any irregularly shaped black or brown spot, having a red, black, or blue coloration on close examination or a bumpy surface, suggests melanoma, and you should report any to your doctor.

The two other kinds of skin cancers are basal cell carcinoma, the least threatening form, characterized by a small raised tumor that often crusts and bleeds, and squamous cell carcinoma, a slow-growing lesion characterized by a firm, red, horn-like appearance.

Lymphatic system

This network of capillaries, thin vessels, valves, ducts, nodes, and organs helps to maintain the body's fluids by filtering, producing, and carrying lymph and other substances throughout your body. Lymph is a fluid somewhat like plasma that, once purified by the lymph nodes, transports fats, proteins, and various blood cells into the blood system. The lymph nodes play an important part in your body's immune reaction by producing a type of white blood cell to fight off infections and by trapping some of the infection-causing agents so they can't spread to other parts of the body.

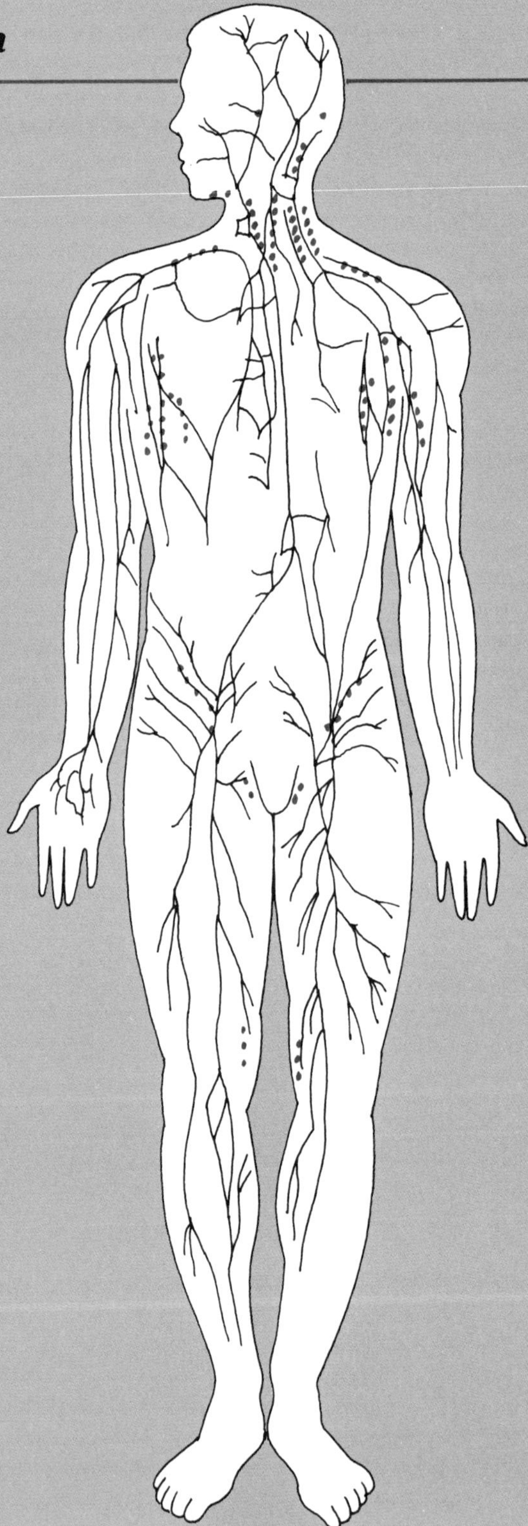

other cells with similar elusive qualities.

Cancer development, then, involves at least two conditions:

- Transformation of a cell through initiation and promotion.
- Some shortcoming in the immune system that lets that cell flourish.

This explains why people given drugs that suppress the immune system—commonly prescribed to recipients of organ transplants to prevent their bodies from rejecting the organs—run a very high risk of cancer.

Cured of cancer?

Most of the 3 million people alive today who have survived cancer are considered cured, while others still have some evidence of cancer. Cured *means that the patient has no evidence of cancer and has the same life expectancy as a person who has never had cancer.*

When is a patient cured of cancer? For most forms of cancer, five years without symptoms following treatment is the accepted time. Some patient can be considered cured after only one year, and others after three years. With some forms of cancer, the period before a patient can be considered cured is longer than five years.

How cancer develops and spreads

Once a cancer cell begins to reproduce, it loses many of the properties restraining the growth of normal cells. For example, one way that a normal cell "knows" when to stop dividing is through interaction with its neighbors. Normal cells exist in neatly arranged sheets and layers. They communicate with one another in several ways: through interactions at boundaries, through substances that pass between cells in the same layer, or through substances transmitted through different layers. Sometimes, a change in the amount of a substance released by one set of cells is interpreted by another set of cells as a signal to start or stop reproducing. As cancer cells grow, they lose not only their restrictions on reproduction; they also lose the ability to interpret the signals sent by other cells.

Thus, as cancer cells proliferate, they shove their neighbors aside, often crushing them. They may also starve their neighbors by using up most of the available nutrient supply. As tumors get even bigger, they may release enzymes that allow them to further invade other cells' territory. These enzymes can also eat holes in nearby blood and lymph vessels, so cells shed by the tumor can enter the circulation and spread (metastasize) to other organs, where they resume the process of proliferation and invasion of normal tissue. In short, cancer spreads by killing off the healthy tissue surrounding it.

The most common cancer targets

The most common cancers in this country are those of the skin, lung, colon and rectum, breast, uterus, and mouth, along with leukemia, which is cancer of the blood cells. Why does cancer have an affinity for some organs more than for others?

One answer is that cancer favors those organs

How cancer invades and kills normal tissues

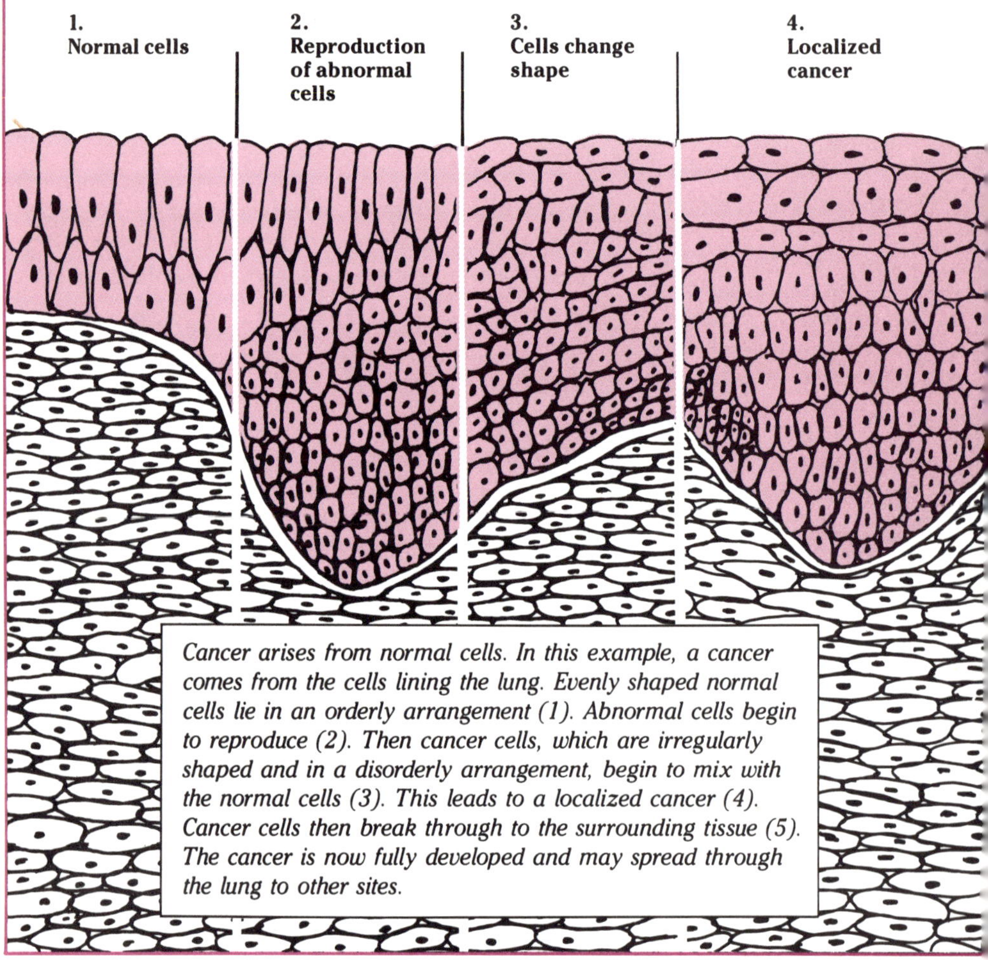

Cancer arises from normal cells. In this example, a cancer comes from the cells lining the lung. Evenly shaped normal cells lie in an orderly arrangement (1). Abnormal cells begin to reproduce (2). Then cancer cells, which are irregularly shaped and in a disorderly arrangement, begin to mix with the normal cells (3). This leads to a localized cancer (4). Cancer cells then break through to the surrounding tissue (5). The cancer is now fully developed and may spread through the lung to other sites.

whose cells grow and divide most rapidly. In the skin, uterus, and digestive tract (colon and rectum), for example, old cells are continually dying and being replaced by new ones. Since cancer is a disease of cell division, it has the best chance of occurring in organs where the rates of cell division are highest.

A second answer is that cancer occurs in those organs most frequently exposed to carcinogenic agents. Again, the skin is a prime example because some part of the skin is often exposed to the ultraviolet light of the sun, which is carcinogenic. Skin cancer therefore occurs most often on the face, head, and neck. The lungs have direct contact with the carcinogens in cigarette smoke, and the more you smoke, the greater your

5.
Developed
cancer

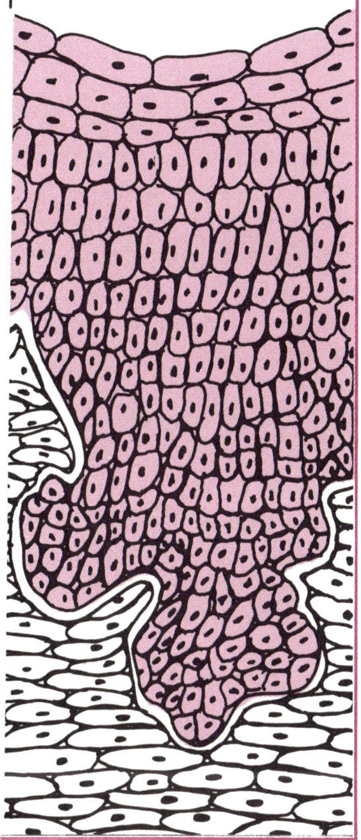

risk of lung cancer. The large intestine is the site of contact with digestive juices called bile acids, which may, under some circumstances, contain promoters or carcinogens.

The third answer draws upon epidemiology, which is the study of diseases in different populations. Through epidemiologic studies, we know, for example, that breast cancer is associated with a high-fat diet, early onset of menstruation, late menopause, and having children late (after age 30) or not at all. What all of this points to is a possible hormonal influence on breast cancer development. From these kinds of studies, some experts conclude that a majority of cancers —more than 70 percent—are caused by life-style factors, including diet, tobacco use, alcohol consumption, and excessive sun exposure. Following is a closer look at the most prevalent forms of cancer in this country.

Skin

There are three kinds of skin cancer: malignant melanoma, basal cell carcinoma, and squamous cell carcinoma. When detected and treated in time, these are among the most curable forms of cancer, but if caught too late, malignant melanoma is one of the most dangerous cancers.

Over 400,000 new cases of skin cancer occur annually, most of which are the highly curable basal and squamous cell carcinomas. All three kinds of skin cancer are related to excessive sun exposure, but malignant melanoma may also run in families. Exposure to substances called polycyclic aromatic hydrocarbons, found in coal tars, soot, asphalt, and lubricating and cutting oils, may add to the risk of squamous cell carcinoma, but this cause isn't nearly as significant as ultraviolet light from the sun.

Lung

Nearly 144,000 new cases of lung cancer occurred in this country in 1985. According to the American Cancer Society, lung cancer may soon surpass breast cancer as the leading cancer killer in women.

Cigarette smoking is the major cause of lung cancer and is estimated to cause 85 percent of lung cancer deaths. People who smoke two or more packs a day have lung cancer death rates that are 15 to 25 times greater than those of nonsmokers. Your risk of contracting lung cancer goes down when you stop smoking.

People who come into contact with asbestos are also at high risk for lung cancer, as are those who work in uranium mines. Smokers who come in contact with asbestos run a risk of lung cancer 50 times greater than the rest of the population. Several other occupational agents contribute to the incidence of lung cancer, including mustard gas, certain kinds of ether, inorganic arsenic, and the minerals chromium and nickel.

Asbestos risk

Family members of people who work with asbestos run higher-than-normal risks of lung cancer just from daily exposure to the dust brought home on clothes. Inhaled asbestos particles produce lung cancer by irritating the lung tissue, which can't dissolve or otherwise remove the particles. Asbestos also has produced cancer of the stomach and intestines.

Genetic structure

Do you resemble your parents? Do your children resemble you? That's because you've inherited your physical traits from your parents, and you've subsequently passed them along to your children. This is also true for individual cells: most cells in your body produce offspring that look pretty much like themselves. A cell's genetic structure regulates this inheritance of characteristics.

Colon and rectum

About 140,000 new cases of colon and rectal cancer occurred in 1985: 95,000 cases in the colon and 40,000 in the rectum. Some 55,000 people died of this form of cancer, a death rate second only to that of lung cancer.

Together, the colon and rectum form the large intestine. The colon is 5 to 6 feet long; the rectum forms the final 5 to 6 inches. Colorectal cancer is most common in people over age 50, making age an important risk factor. Inherited risks may exist, too: small colon growths called polyps appear more frequently in some families and carry with them an extremely high risk of subsequent colon cancer. People who have had Crohn's disease, a chronic inflammation of the lower section of the small intestine, or prolonged, extensive ulcerative colitis (chronic inflammation of the large intestine) are also highly vulnerable to colorectal cancer.

A high-fiber, low-fat diet may protect you from colorectal cancer. The evidence is especially good for fiber: in those people whose diets are high in both fat and fiber, the incidence of colorectal cancer is relatively low, although doctors are still not sure why.

Breast

Breast cancer is the leading cancer killer in women. In 1985, some 120,000 new cases occurred, and about 40,000 women will die of it. The American Cancer Society estimates that about 1 out of every 11 women will develop breast cancer.

Hormones apparently play a role in stimulating breast cancer development. Women who menstruate early, reach menopause late, and who take replacement estrogen hormones are at high risk for breast cancer because they're exposed to certain hormones longer than other women. A high-fat diet may further

Cancer by site and sex

These figures provide a breakdown by site and sex for the major kinds of cancer. As you can see, the most prevalent cancers for men are of the lung, prostate, and colon and rectum. For women, the most prevalent cancers are of the breast, colon and rectum, and uterus.

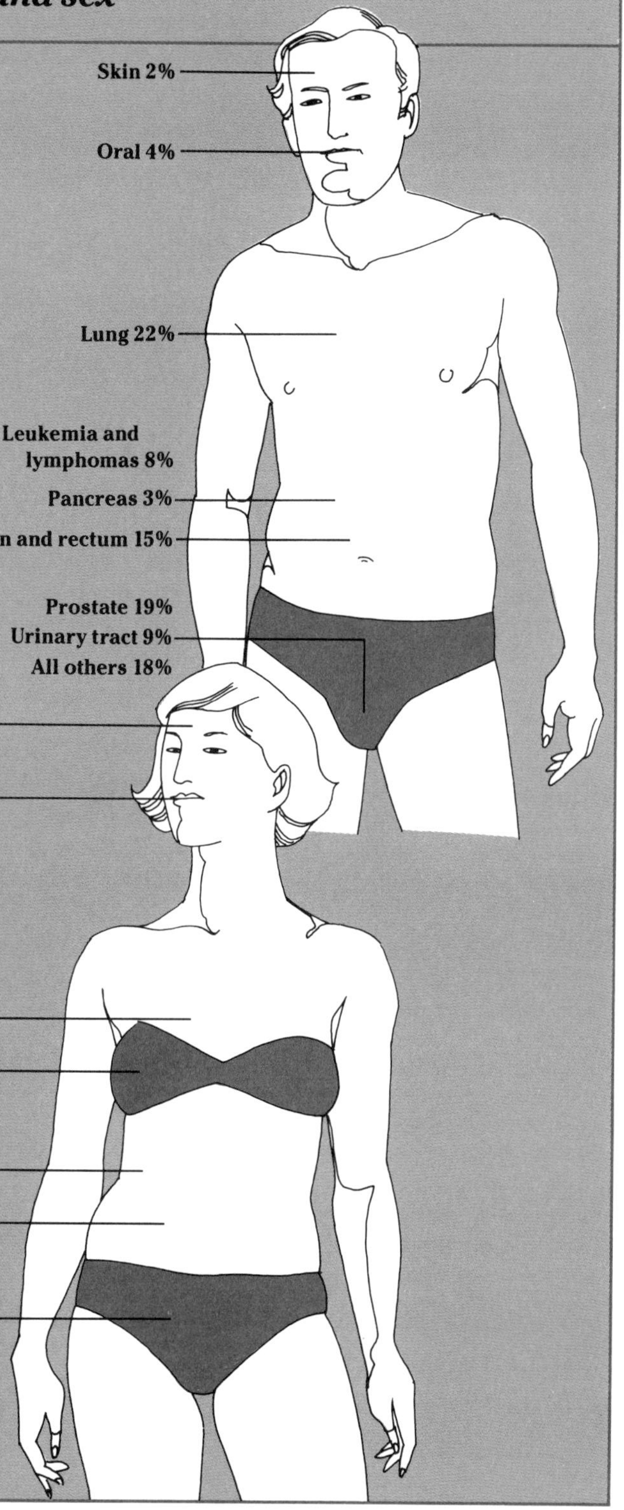

stimulate the effects of these hormones, although this isn't yet proven. Other risks include family history:

- If you're a woman whose mother or sister has had breast cancer, your chances of getting it are doubled.
- If both your sister and mother have had breast cancer, your chances are 6 times greater.

Your chances are also higher:

- If you're obese.
- If you had your first child after age 30.
- If you've already had cancer in one breast.
- If you have a history of benign fibrocystic breast disease.

Uterus

The uterus has two portions: the cervix, or opening, and the corpus, also known as the body or the womb. The corpus has two layers: the inner layer, or endometrium, and the outer layer, or myometrium. Cancers can occur in either the cervix or the endometrium.

About 52,000 new cases of uterine cancer occurred in 1985: 37,000 in the endometrium and 15,000 in the cervix.

Cervical cancer in this country has been declining steadily for the past 30 years because of the development of the Pap smear, a test developed to encourage early detection of cervical cancer. No one cause of cervical cancer has been identified, but some of the risk factors include multiple sex partners, early age of first intercourse, smoking, and type of contraception used (more cervical cancer is seen in women who use birth-control pills).

Endometrial cancer is the third most common cancer in American women, after skin and breast cancers. It shares some risk factors with breast cancer:

- Obesity.
- Few or no children.
- Onset of menstruation at an early age.
- Late menopause.

As with breast cancer, endometrial cancer may be related to hormone imbalances. Women on certain forms of the Pill seem to be protected from endometrial cancer.

Acute and chronic leukemia

Leukemia can be acute or chronic.

Acute leukemia develops rapidly. If left untreated, it kills within a few months. Fortunately, current treatment methods permit most acute leukemia patients to survive for several years. In adults, the most common form of leukemia is an acute leukemia called acute nonlymphocytic leukemia (ANL).

Chronic leukemia develops more slowly. Even if it's not treated, its victims can live for years, because the cancer cells grow slowly.

The symptoms for each kind of leukemia are similar: fatigue, easy bruising, infection, fever. With chronic leukemia, however, they're more subtle and take longer to develop.

Controlling the risks

You can control many of the risks associated with the major forms of cancer, with the possible exception of leukemia. Often you can greatly lower your cancer risk by making some changes in your life-style. In the next chapter, we'll examine some of the main cancer causes and what you can do about them.

Essential differences between benign and malignant tumors

Technically, the word *tumor* refers to any abnormal growth, not just cancer. Of the many different kinds of tumors, only a small fraction are cancerous. What's the difference?

Benign tumor cells grow faster than normal cells, but slower than malignant cells. They don't spread, and they don't invade surrounding or underlying tissue, as do malignant tumor cells. Because they don't spread, benign tumors are cured when removed, but if they're not removed in time, some benign tumors may become malignant.

Malignant tumors are made up of rapidly growing abnormal cells that can spread to other parts of the body and will destroy normal cells in surrounding tissue.

This chart summarizes some of the major differences between benign and malignant tumors.

Characteristic	Benign	Malignant
Growth	Slow expansion; push aside surrounding tissue but don't invade	Rapid invasion of surrounding tissues, extending in all directions
Recurrence	When removed surgically, don't recur	When removed surgically, frequently recur due to infiltration into surrounding tissues
Appearance	Cells closely resemble those of tissue of origin	Cells vary abnormally from those of tissue of origin
Tissue destruction	Minimal	Extensive due to infiltration and spreading
Spread	Don't spread; remain localized	Spread through blood and/or lymph systems; establish secondary tumors
Effect on body	Usually don't kill but may obstruct vital organs, exert pressure, produce excess hormones. Can become malignant	Loss of weight, weakness, anemia. Always kill if not removed surgically or treated promptly before they spread

Mouth

The most common oral cancer sites are the lips, tongue, floor of the mouth, soft palate, tonsils, salivary glands, and back of the throat. However, cancer may develop in any part of the oral cavity. According to the American Cancer Society, 29,000 new cases of oral cancer occurred in 1985, mostly in men over age 40. Tobacco use is the primary risk factor: not only smoking, but tobacco chewing and even "snuff dipping," which consists of holding a pinch of finely ground tobacco between your gum and your cheek. This custom is growing among people who mistakenly believe they can lower their risk of cancer while indulging in some form of tobacco use. In fact, snuff dipping can cause cancers of the gum and cheek lining.

Heavy alcohol consumption (more than seven drinks a week) has also been related to oral cancer, but since heavy drinkers often smoke, separating the effects of the two is difficult. Heavy drinkers run about double the normal risk of mouth and throat cancer. If you smoke *and* drink, your risk is greater than you'd expect from simply adding the two factors together.

Certain workers seem to be at higher risk for oral cancer, including bartenders, waiters and waitresses, printers, farmers, sailors, outdoor workers, electronics workers, leather workers, and paper manufacturers. Nevertheless, the National Cancer Institute maintains that quitting cigarettes, pipes, and snuff would drastically reduce the incidence of cancers of the mouth and throat.

Cancer and the Pill

Birth-control pills developed a reputation as carcinogens because of early animal studies done with one of the Pill's hormone ingredients. These studies showed that laboratory animals ran an increased risk of tumors of the cervix, vagina, and liver, as well as the breast. Human studies conducted since then, however, haven't borne this out. The most important findings in humans are:

- *The Pill might place you at higher risk for breast cancer* if you already *have a history of breast cysts.*
- *Taking the Pill may prevent you from developing breast cysts if you don't have them already.*
- *The Pill might place you at a slightly higher than normal risk of some kinds of liver tumors.*

Leukemia

About 25,000 new cases of leukemia occurred in 1985. The four different kinds of leukemia together account for only 5 percent of the overall cancer incidence in the United States, but for about 45 percent—nearly half—of the cancer in children.

White blood cells, part of your immune system, normally fight infections and carry oxygen to tissues. With leukemia, abnormal white blood cells enter the circulation and prevent the healthy white blood cells from doing their jobs. People with leukemia, therefore, run a very high risk of infections and anemia.

Causes for the different kinds of leukemia vary. The best-known causes include genetic predisposition (tendency), malfunction of the immune system, and exposure to environmental factors, such as chemicals, radiation, and viruses.

2 Does everything cause cancer?

You do have choices

The two major causes of cancer are diet and tobacco. You can avoid the riskiest foods and food additives if you try, and you can control your use of tobacco. Work and environmental pollutants pose problems for some people. To begin, find out which substances are risky and then decide what you can do for yourself. This chapter will help you.

Despite all the cancer publicity, everything doesn't cause cancer, and you can avoid most of the things that do. The first two discussed here, diet and cigarettes, together account for about 65 percent—just about two-thirds—of all the cancer that occurs in this country.

The fears over what causes cancer have been exaggerated. Our society does rely heavily on synthetic compounds, and these aren't always tested as thoroughly as they should be before they're introduced to the public. Based on current knowledge, however, only a small fraction of those chemicals are thought to cause cancer, and they contribute minimally to the total cancer risk most Americans face. Of the approximately 50,000 known chemicals, roughly 7,000 have been tested for carcinogenicity, mostly because they were suspicious. Of those 7,000, about 700 to 800—approximately 10 percent—can cause cancer.

Today, government agencies regulate the use of identified carcinogens in our food, air, water, and workplaces. This doesn't mean they've been banned entirely: in some cases, this simply hasn't been practical. Saccharin, for example, causes bladder cancer in laboratory animals. Officials considered banning it from our food supply, as they did cyclamates a few years earlier, but public pressure convinced them not to do so. In this case, the benefits from having saccharin available looked stronger than the risk that it might cause cancer in some people.

A similar case exists with the drug reserpine, an important part of therapy for patients with high blood pressure. It can cause tumors in laboratory animals, but its effect on people is still in question. Most doctors feel that reserpine's importance in controlling high blood pressure in some patients outweighs its risk.

The best way for you to lower your cancer risk is to decrease your exposure to those agents whose risks don't outweigh their benefits. Some have no benefits at all, like cigarettes. Others are naturally occurring parts of the environment and can't be avoided entirely, like sunlight. Still others can remain enjoyable parts of our lives if used in moderation, like certain foods.

Diet

One of the most heated controversies in cancer research centers on the role of diet in causing, preventing, and treating cancer. According to the National Cancer Institute, diet causes up to 35 percent of all the cancers seen in this country—even more than that caused by cigarettes. More specifically, eating habits are held responsible for 60 percent of the cancer in women, and 40 percent of the cancer in men.

High-fiber foods and cancer

People have been saying it for years—roughage is good for you—and they were right. Today, we usually refer to roughage as "fiber." High-fiber foods are believed to help prevent some forms of cancer. Such foods include celery, carrots, pears, apples, lettuce, bran cereal, and whole-grain breads and pasta.

Some of the nutrients and foods that may treat or prevent cancer include:

- vitamin A
- vitamin C
- vitamin E
- fiber-rich foods.

Some of the foods and food additives thought to raise cancer risk include:

- high-fat foods
- certain food dyes
- nitrites and nitrates (food preservatives)
- alcohol.

Questions remain about these substances:

- saccharin and cyclamates
- BHA and BHT (food preservatives)
- pesticides
- hormone residues in meats.

Vitamins

Vitamins may help fight some cancers by decreasing the formation of carcinogenic waste products in the cell. Your body can generally dispose of these wastes without problems, but an adequate vitamin supply in your diet gives you an extra margin of safety.

Scientists first started examining the role of vitamins in cancer prevention when they found that cancer incidence is low among groups of people whose diets are high in vitamins A, C, and E. For example, in one Norwegian study of 8,000 men, both smokers and nonsmokers, lung cancer rates were lowest among those men who consumed the most Vitamin A. Similar studies done in other countries have had similar results.

Diet and cancer

To lower your cancer risk, decrease your exposure to risky agents. Since some of these agents are in food, you may wonder how you should plan what you eat. The old rule of thumb will still work very well: vary your diet and eat in moderation. Choose from the four basic food groups and emphasize complex carbohydrates and fiber over fatty foods.

Every day, a certain amount of your food should come from each of the four basic food groups.

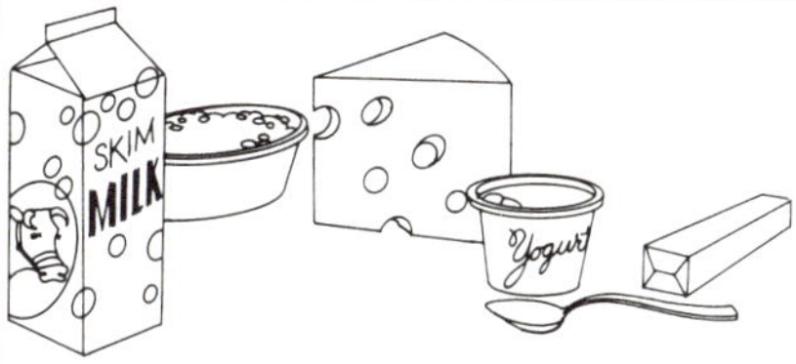

Milk group
Milk and everything made from it, such as cheese, ice cream, and yogurt. If you're watching your fat intake, concentrate on low-fat or skimmed milk, cheeses like cottage cheese and ricotta made from low-fat milk, and yogurt.

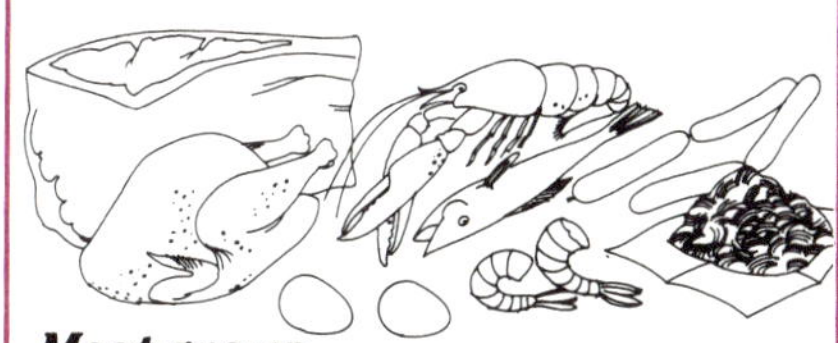

Meat group
Includes beef and other meats, fish, poultry, and eggs. If you're watching your fat intake, eat more chicken and turkey (remove the skin), rabbit, and fish.

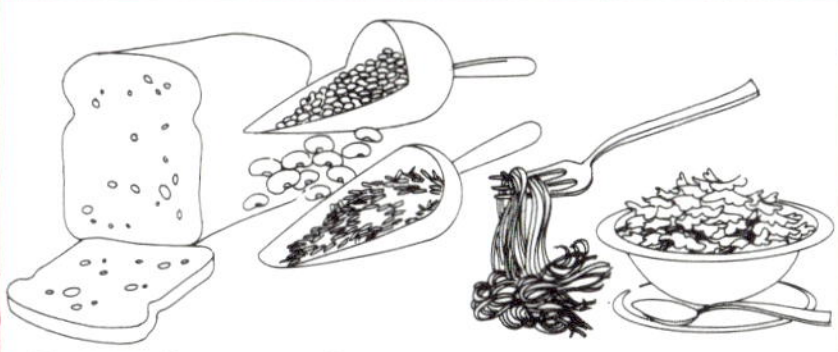

Bread-cereal group
If you're increasing your intake of fiber, bread and cereals are important—provided you avoid foods made with all-purpose flour. So you'll want whole-grain bread and pasta and foods like brown rice, barley, bulgur, millet, and buckwheat.

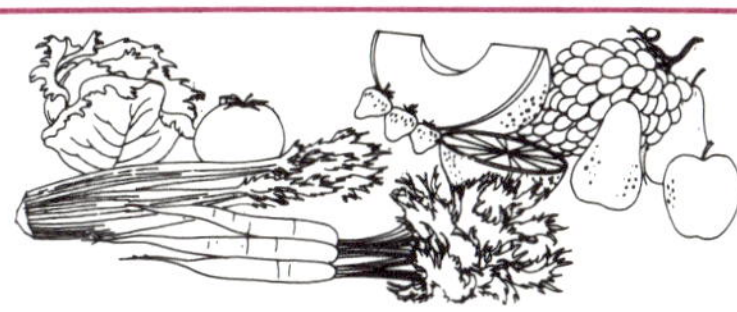

Fruit-vegetable group
If you're watching your fiber intake, greatly increase the number and variety of fruits and vegetables you eat. Most are good fiber sources, and some vegetables may contain anticancer factors. Among these are cabbage, kohlrabi, broccoli, cauliflower, and Brussels sprouts.

Fiber

Fiber is a necessary part of our diet with several important functions, even though it passes through the digestive tract largely unchanged. It draws water into the digestive tract, softening the tract's contents and thus facilitating digestion and elimination; helps maintain the health of the digestive tract; may help lower blood cholesterol; and helps prevent colon cancer. Fiber is thought to lower the cancer risk by hastening the passage of food through the digestive tract, decreasing the amount of time cells in the tract are exposed to any cancer-causing agents in the food. It also indirectly decreases the level of potentially carcinogenic substances produced by the body. When dietary fiber is low, the body manufactures large quantities of bile acids that are released into the digestive tract to aid digestion. These bile acids may contain a compound that causes DNA mutation in the cells of the colon, thus starting the cancer process. A diet that includes enough fiber inhibits production of these bile acids. The presence of fiber also encourages the growth of beneficial gut bacteria, while its absence may allow dangerous bacteria to proliferate.

Excessive fat

A high-fat diet has been linked to cancer of the breast, colon, uterus, and prostate gland. According to one theory, this kind of diet, consumed by the majority of Americans, may stimulate hormone production, which in turn affects cell metabolism and may place cells at greater risk of becoming cancerous. A second theory states that a large intake of fat promotes the release of bile acids. A high-fat diet may encourage the growth of some kinds of digestive tract bacteria that manufacture carcinogens. Processed fats in much of our food may contribute to the problem by making cells more vulnerable to attack by free radicals, which are digestive by-products that, when they accumulate, may cause DNA mutations.

Limit your fat intake

Follow these guidelines to limit your fat intake:

- *Limit the size of meat portions—a total of 6 ounces a day is adequate for most people. Choose lean meats rather than those that are fatty, and limit your use of sausage and luncheon meats.*
- *Trim fat from meat and skin from poultry.*
- *Substitute low-fat dairy products for those high in fat. Use skim milk instead of whole milk, and use nonfat powdered milk in baking. Use low-fat yogurt or imitation sour cream instead of real sour cream, and try evaporated skim milk in recipes that call for heavy cream. Use low-fat cheeses, such as cottage cheese, part-skim mozzarella, or ricotta. Avoid such high-fat cheeses as cheddar, cream, brie, and Swiss.*
- *Read labels carefully and avoid foods high in fat.*
- *Limit fat in cooking, and avoid fried foods. Bake or broil meat, and use a rack in the pan when cooking meats to allow fat to drip out. When possible, poach food in water or broth rather than sautéing it, and use nonstick pans to limit the need for fat in cooking. Steam vegetables quickly instead of cooking them with fat.*
- *Use only small amounts of regular salad dressings.*
- *Adjust baked-good recipes by using one-half to three-fourths the amount of fat recommended.*
- *Limit your intake of nuts and seeds—they're naturally high in fat.*

Choose low-fat, high-nutrient snacks, such as fresh fruit, raw vegetables, popcorn, and whole-grain, low-fat crackers.

Major cancer risk factors

Knowing some of the factors that have been linked to cancer will help you protect yourself. Some of these factors, like diet, are complicated; others, like smoking, aren't. You can learn about even the more complicated aspects of diet in this chapter. This chart shows the major cancer risk factors and their contributions to the total U.S. cancer incidence. (The factors don't total 100% because some haven't been isolated.)

Risk factor	Estimated total incidence
Diet	35%
Tobacco	30%
Viruses	5%
Occupation	4%
Alcohol	3%
Excess sunshine	3%
Environmental pollution	2%
Medicine and medical procedures	1%
Food additives	1% or less

Food dyes, preservatives, and pesticides

The most heated debate concerning food and cancer concentrates on the presence of alleged carcinogens in our food. "Experts" noisily argue whether pesticides, food dyes, and preservatives are dangerous chemicals that should be banned from our food supply or are beneficial substances that enhance the safety and palatability of our food. As with any controversy, the truth is hard to isolate. A closer look at two of these substances, nitrites and nitrates, helps illustrate the complexities involved.

Nitrites and nitrates are added to foods such as packaged meats to prevent the growth of an organism called *Clostridium botulinum*. If allowed to grow unchecked, *Clostridium botulinum* would cause botulism, a fatal disease. The nitrites and nitrates also prevent the growth of salmonella, which can cause sometimes-fatal food poisoning. Finally, nitrites and nitrates preserve the pink color characteristic of bologna, salami, ham, and similar products. But despite their role in our food supply, once in the body, nitrites and nitrates are converted by our digestive acids into substances called nitrosamines, which are carcinogenic.

Pesticides in the food you eat

Pesticides and other chemicals can enter your body in several ways. One of the most direct is illustrated here.

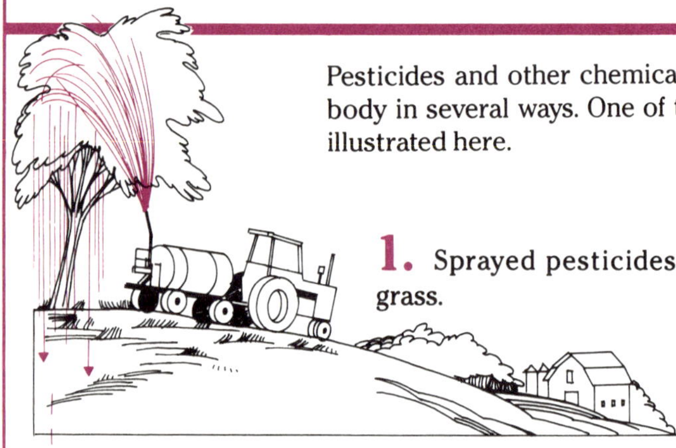

1. Sprayed pesticides fall on grass.

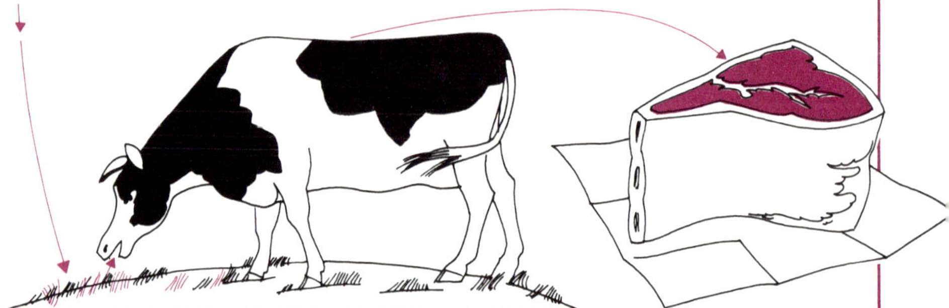

2. Cattle eat the grass, and the pesticides settle in the animals' fat.

3. The cattle are slaughtered, and you eat the chemicals in the meat.

Many people feel that, no matter how beneficial these additives may be, they should be removed from our food if they cause cancer. Others argue that without the added nitrites and nitrates, these convenience foods would have to come off the market. Adding to this complexity is the interesting discovery that Vitamin C that is eaten with foods containing nitrites or nitrates combines with these substances and prevents the formation of nitrosamines. For now, then, you should cut back on your eating of foods with added nitrites and nitrates and, when you do eat them, have an orange, or orange juice, or a green, leafy vegetable.

Food industry advocates argue that most of the chemicals added to our food are safe. For example, they claim that the food dyes currently used aren't believed to be carcinogenic, and point out that dyes with known cancer-causing effects already have been banned from our food supply. But according to consumer advocates, our food still contains dozens of coloring agents and other additives that, while perhaps not proven carcinogens, certainly haven't been proven safe.

Along with dyes and preservatives, hormones and pesticides are controversial. Cattle are routinely given hormones to speed their growth. So are chickens. Some of these hormones, particularly diethylstilbestrol (DES), are now known to be human carcinogens, and in 1979 the Food and Drug Administration (FDA) banned DES's use. Some ranchers have ignored that ban, and consumers cannot be certain that their meat is free from DES. What's more, the ban on DES hasn't prevented farmers from giving their animals similar hormones, which may ultimately prove to be just as harmful.

More about cigarettes

Cigarettes have been linked to several diseases other than cancer, including heart disease, high blood pressure, and stomach ailments. They increase your need for nutrients like Vitamin C, and if you're a pregnant woman who smokes, your baby may be born smaller and run a greater risk of dying shortly after birth.

Cigarettes

According to the World Health Organization, we'll see a global epidemic of lung cancer by the end of this century. In China and India, the world's two most densely populated countries, one-quarter to one-third of the men are addicted to cigarettes by the time they reach age 18. In this country, as many as two-thirds of the men under age 40 have been addicted to cigarettes at one time. Fortunately, these numbers have declined as researchers have linked cigarettes with so many health problems.

Passive smoking hazards

Nonsmokers who breathe the smoke of smokers' cigarettes may be in danger. Such smoking is known as "passive" smoking. Recent studies indicate an increased risk of lung cancer among the nonsmoking wives of cigarette smokers. Other studies, however, have failed to find any risk for such passive smokers, and the question has not yet been resolved.

Nevertheless, in 1985, 126,000 Americans died of lung cancer. That represents about one-third of all the cancer deaths for that year. Lung cancer is the fastest-rising cancer in women, possibly because more women and teenage girls are smoking: in 1960, 6,000 women died of lung cancer, while in 1980 it killed 27,000 women. That's an increase of more than 400 percent! Its incidence in men is also rising, but not as fast.

Lung cancer is one of the deadliest forms of cancer: less than one-tenth of all lung cancers are curable by the time they're detected. Why? Tumors of the lung and respiratory tract are "clinically silent." That is, they may show no symptoms until they've advanced too far to be cured. One expert estimates that 200,000 Americans may currently have undetected respiratory tumors.

The symptoms of lung cancer include:

- coughing
- pain in the chest, back, and shoulder blades
- bad breath
- pneumonia: cough, fever, chills, malaise, and loss of appetite.

The lung tumor that grows large enough can affect the blood supply to the heart. Certain kinds of lung tumors compress the spinal nerves, causing pain in the arm and shoulder and deterioration of the muscles in the arm and hand. As the tumor grows even bigger, it may erode ribs and vertebrae, leading to bone pain.

Tobacco isn't the only cause of lung cancer, but it can amplify the effects of other causes. Smokers who work with asbestos, for example, run a far greater risk of lung cancer than do nonsmokers working with the same substance.

As if this weren't bad enough, evidence links cigarettes with other forms of cancer. They've been associated with cancers of the lip, mouth, tongue, larynx, pharynx, esophagus, bladder, pancreas, kidney, stomach, and, possibly, the cervix. According to the National Cancer Institute, cigarette smokers have an

A growing cancerous tumor can destroy a lung's ability to function. Growth of the tumor cuts off blood flow to the lung and blocks the lung's airway. Deprived of blood and oxygen, lung tissue dies.

Cancer invasion of a lung

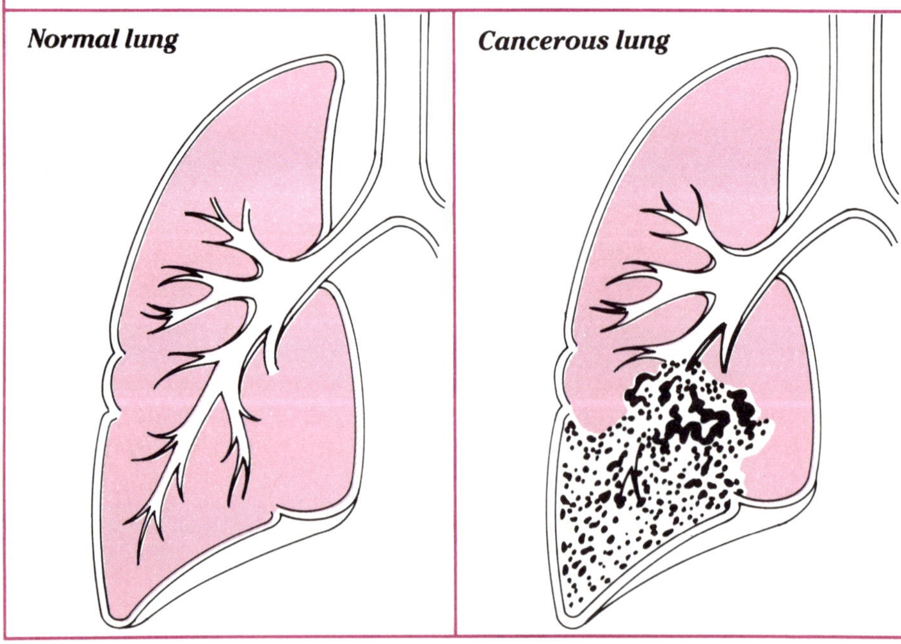

Giving up cigarettes

If you smoke, quitting is about the best thing you can do toward better health and longer life. Dedicate yourself to quitting: use all your imagination and all your willpower. The following are only some of the methods other smokers have used to quit.

• Hypnosis. Many have quit with the help of hypnosis. Ask your doctor for an opinion and a recommendation.

• Aversion therapy. In aversion therapy you'll associate an unpleasant experience, such as a strong unpleasant odor, with smoking. Again, ask your doctor for an opinion and recommendation.

• Reason with yourself. Write down your reasons for wanting to stop smoking and your reasons for wanting to continue smoking. Each night, repeat at least 10 times the reason to quit that means the most to you—and do the same each time you reach for a cigarette. Do you really want it?

• Cutting down to none. Many people have found that the best way to quit is to gradually cut the number of cigarettes they smoke to one a day—and then to eliminate that one. You can help yourself cut down by keeping a record of the cigarettes you smoke: when, where, and why you smoke each one. Wrap a piece of paper around your package of cigarettes, and write down the information each time you take a cigarette. Make a special note of the cigarettes that are most important to you (those immediately after meals, for example), the ones that are least important (perhaps the one smoked while waiting for the bus), and the one that tasted especially good (the first one of the day, perhaps). Establish a number of cigarettes for each day, and then eliminate one cigarette each day—or each week. You can choose to begin by eliminating the cigarette that you desired least or the one you desired most.

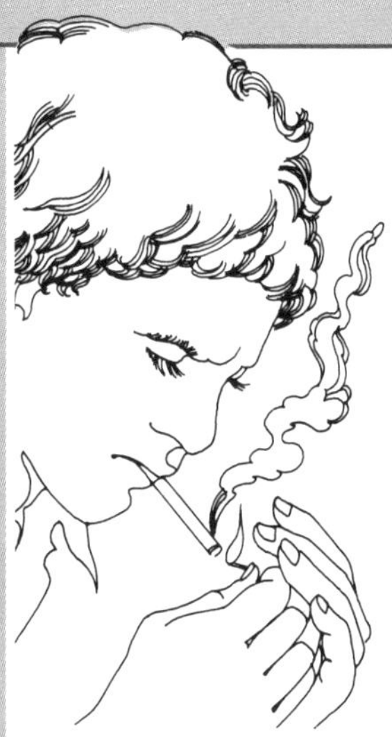

Bad news

Virtually all lung cancers are linked to smoking, and fewer than one-tenth are curable. Don't smoke.

• Quitting cold. Quitting "cold turkey" works for many people. Choose a day—give yourself plenty of time but no more than five or six weeks—and when the day comes, quit. Plan plenty of activities for the chosen day.

• Get help. To quit, you may want to join a group. Several organizations specialize in helping smokers quit. The American Cancer Society has some very helpful material on the benefits of giving up cigarettes. They also conduct smoke withdrawal programs. If the society doesn't have a branch near you, write to its national headquarters: 777 Third Avenue, New York, NY 10017.

Don't be discouraged if you don't successfully quit the first time you try. Keep trying—the results are worth it.

overall cancer risk double that of nonsmokers. In heavy smokers (more than one pack a day), the risk may be three or four times that of nonsmokers. The more you smoke, the greater your cancer risk, and if you smoke while drinking alcohol, your risk of certain cancers is increased even more. But when you quit, your chances of getting cancer decrease.

If you think you can cut your risk of cancer by switching to a cigar or pipe, think again. Tobacco in almost any form causes cancer; its smoke contains nearly 4,000 substances that act as initiators, promoters, and carcinogens. Snuff and chewing tobacco will increase your risk of cancer of the mouth and throat.

The evidence is clear: if you want to lower your cancer risk, don't smoke!

Alcohol, tobacco, and cancer

The heavy use of alcohol, especially when accompanied by cigarette smoking or smokeless tobacco, increases the risk of cancers of the mouth, larynx, throat, esophagus, and liver.

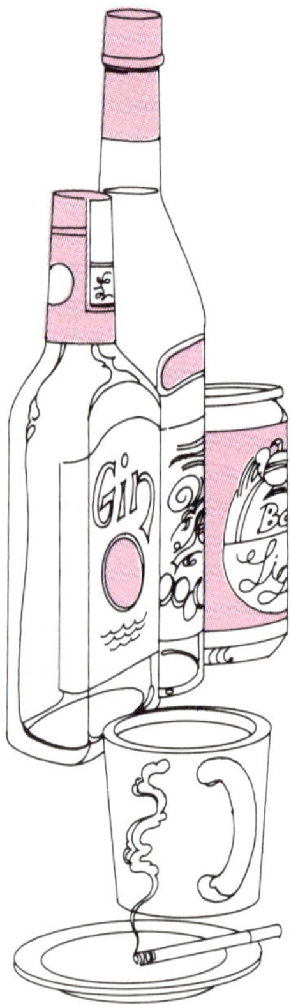

Alcohol

According to the National Cancer Institute, consumption of alcoholic beverages increases the risk of cancer of the mouth, pharynx, larynx, and esophagus. This may be due not only to the alcohol itself, but to the effects of some of the added flavorings and substances produced during fermentation, which may act with the alcohol as co-carcinogens. Since many heavy drinkers also smoke, isolating the effects of alcohol from those of tobacco is difficult, but evidence suggests that heavy alcohol consumption directly increases the risk of esophageal cancer. Since many heavy drinkers don't eat well, the lack of protective nutrients may further increase their cancer risk.

Cyclamates and saccharin

Cyclamates, artificial sweeteners that were popular in the 1960s, have been banned in this country since 1969, when they were found to cause bladder cancer in laboratory animals. Saccharin is also thought to be a promoter and a weak carcinogen, but studies in diabetics who have been long-term saccharin users haven't revealed a higher cancer incidence over the rest of the population. The slight risk of developing cancer seems to be worth the benefits of saccharin for the millions of diabetics who need it and the many millions more who are watching their weight.

The anticancer diet

No doubt you've found some of this information surprising, some of it frightening, and much of it confusing. How can we make sense of all the different opinions and conflicting evidence we hear? How can we deal with the risks to our long-term health? The following diet guidelines, recommended by the American Cancer Society, will not only lower your risk of cancer but may help you avoid other diseases as well.

Cruciferous vegetables
Cruciferous vegetables have flowers with four leaves in the pattern of a cross. Among these vegetables are cabbage, broccoli, Brussels sprouts, kohlrabi, and cauliflower. These vegetables may help prevent certain cancers from developing. Research is in progress to determine how.

1. Avoid obesity. People who are 40 percent or greater overweight run an increased risk of colon, breast, and uterine cancers. Exercise is a great way to burn calories and control appetite; try to add 20 minutes of moderate exercise, like walking, to your daily routine. To cut calories follow the next guideline.

2. Cut down on total fat intake. Only 30 percent of your daily calories should come from fat; if you're average, your current intake is about 40 percent. Ounce for ounce, fat has more than twice the calories of protein or carbohydrates. And, as mentioned earlier, high-fat foods increase the risk of several kinds of cancer. By cutting down on fat, you'll reduce both your weight and your cancer risk.

3. Eat more high-fiber foods. Not only do they lower your risk of colon cancer, high-fiber foods make good substitutes for fatty foods because they absorb water in the digestive tract and help you feel full. Fresh apples, pears, melons, strawberries, peas, beans, carrots, broccoli, and whole grain breads and cereals are all good sources of dietary fiber.

4. Include foods rich in vitamins A and C in your daily diet. For Vitamin A, choose dark green and deep yellow fruits and vegetables, such as carrots, spinach, yams, peaches, and apricots. For Vitamin C, oranges, grapefruits, strawberries, and red and green peppers are good sources.

5. Include vegetables such as cabbage, broccoli, Brussels sprouts, and cauliflower in your diet; such foods may help prevent the development of certain cancers. Research is now in progress to determine what is in these foods that may protect against cancer.

6. Avoid salt-cured, smoked, and nitrite-cured foods. In parts of the world where salt-cured and smoked foods are eaten frequently, the incidence of cancer of the stomach and esophagus is greater. The role of nitrites and nitrates in cancer development may be relatively minor, but they do represent an additional risk you can easily avoid. Besides, the meats

Vitamins A and C

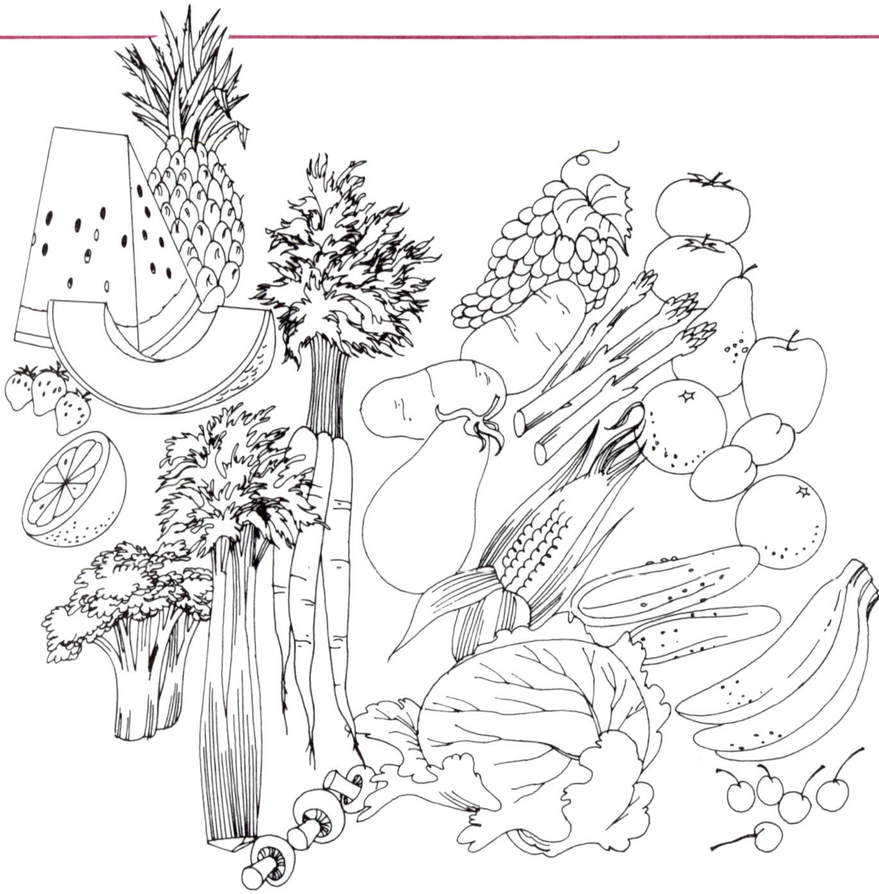

Eating foods high in vitamins A and C has been associated with lower rates of some cancers. Certain fruits and vegetables are the best sources of these vitamins. Follow these guidelines:

- *Eat plenty of dark green and deep yellow or red fruits and vegetables. These include apricots, cantaloupe, nectarines, papayas, and watermelon; broccoli, carrots, sweet potatoes, winter squash, and all dark leafy vegetables such as spinach and chard.*
- *Vitamin C–rich fruits include cantaloupe, grapefruit, oranges, and strawberries. The best vegetable sources of Vitamin C are broccoli, collard and turnip greens, peppers, and tomato juice.*
- *Try eating these vegetables raw or cooked quickly by either steaming or stir-frying. They'll stay crisper and more flavorful, and fewer of their nutrients will be destroyed.*
- *Try salads made of dark greens such as spinach or nonleafy vegetables such as green peppers, carrots, broccoli, tomatoes, and cauliflower.*
- *Marinate cut-up vegetables in a container with lemon juice or vinegar, herbs, and spices. Serve them at meals or as snacks.*
- *Increase the amount of vegetables in meat-vegetable casseroles while decreasing the amount of meat.*
- *Eat fruit instead of candy or cookies.*
- *Drink fruit juices instead of coffee, tea, or soda.*

they're added to are often salted or smoked as well. If you must eat these foods, have a citrus fruit, citrus juice, or tomato juice along with them: all are high in Vitamin C.

7. If you drink alcohol, do so in moderation.

Edible soybeans
You probably think of soybeans as food for cattle, but they're high in protein, so scientists have worked hard to develop more palatable kinds. Today you can buy or grow edible soybeans that taste like lima beans. These edible soybeans grow well in cool northern climates.

Canned or dried?
You can buy beans canned or dried. Canned beans are convenient, but dried beans are even more economical.

Anticancer meals

A nutritious, anticancer diet needn't be boring, tasteless, or inflexible. Indeed, learning about healthful foods and healthful ways to prepare foods will introduce you to the wide variety of available vegetables and grains. The following are only a few suggestions.

- Use legumes. Legumes—dried beans and peas—are quite popular in many foreign countries, but many Americans consume them infrequently. A good source of protein, iron, magnesium, zinc, and several B vitamins, legumes can make a valuable contribution to your diet. They're also high in fiber. Extra servings of legumes can help compensate for nutrients lost with smaller meat portions. What's more, legumes are inexpensive and easy to cook.

Nutrition facts

Remember these facts about nutrition when planning meals:

Whole grains, legumes, and dairy products provide protein without meat.

Cooking vegetables by steaming is quick, destroys fewer vitamins than do other methods, and adds no fat.

Fruits make excellent desserts. Strawberries, for example, are high in Vitamin C and lower in calories and fat than many typical desserts.

Whole grain foods—like popcorn or low-fat crackers—are good for snacks—they provide more nutrients and fewer calories than potato chips or pretzels.

Whole grains are best for breakfast, too. Select cereals—whether ready-to-eat or cooked—that have whole grain products first in the list of ingredients. Shredded wheat is an example of a whole grain cereal.

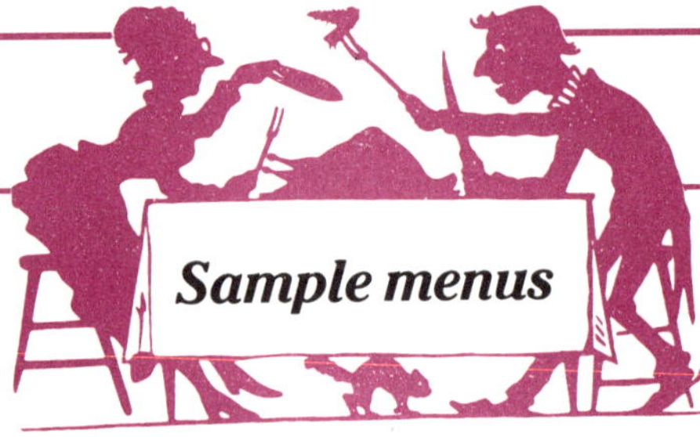

Sample menus

These two menus are based on the anticancer tips in this book. They're designed to provide an average of 1,600 daily calories—enough for the sedentary life-style of many Americans. These are only samples, of course; when planning your own menus, you'll want to consider your personal likes and dislikes (and those of family members), the scheduling of your meals, your cooking style, the location of your meals, and other factors. However, you can accommodate such matters while still meeting nutritional needs and following the guidelines suggested to reduce the risk of cancer.

Breakfast	**Breakfast**
3/4 cup ready-to-eat whole grain cereal with 1/2 cup cantaloupe and 1/2 cup skim or low-fat milk	2 whole wheat pancakes, each spread with 1/4 cup cottage cheese and sprinkled with cinnamon
Lunch	**Lunch**
Small wedge of lettuce, 1/2 cup carrots, 1/4 cup raw cauliflower and 1/2 cup garbanzo or kidney beans with 2 tablespoons of regular salad dressing 6 whole grain rye wafers	Chicken sandwich (3 ounces chicken with 1 tablespoon mayonnaise on 2 slices whole-wheat bread) 1 cup skim milk
Dinner	**Dinner**
6 ounces chicken or veal, cooked with lemon and parsley 1 cup whole wheat noodles with 1 1/2 teaspoons margarine 3/4 cup tomato and basil salad	Tabouli (bulgur, parsley, tomato, garbanzo beans, and oil) Shish kebab made with 3 ounces marinated chicken or lean beef, pork, or lamb; 1/2 green pepper, and 1/2 cup tomato and onion
Evening snack 1 bran muffin	

Dried beans, such as kidney, lima, garbanzo, pinto, and navy, and lentils can be combined with other ingredients in soups, salads, and stews. You can serve them alone flavored with herbs and other seasonings, or you can puree them and make them into sandwich spreads and dips.

Garbanzos?
Unfamiliar with garbanzo beans? Perhaps you know them by their other name—chick peas. And if you don't know them at all, introduce yourself.

Bulgur wheat
Bulgur (the name is Turkish) is whole wheat that has been steamed, dried, and cracked for quicker cooking. It's a fine substitute for rice or potatoes.

• Experiment with parsley. Small amounts of parsley used as seasoning don't contribute much to your diet, but when used in larger quantities, parsley contributes many nutrients.

• Use whole-wheat flour. Substitute whole-wheat flour in your favorite recipes and try reducing the amount of fat used, too.

• Use whole grains. Use whole-wheat flour instead of all-purpose flour in recipes for baked goods. One cup of finely milled whole wheat flour (or ⅞ if coarsely ground) substitutes for one cup of all-purpose flour. Check the ingredients on ready-made bread to make sure the first ingredient listed—the one present in the largest amount—is whole grain flour. Use brown (unpolished) rice in place of white (polished) rice. Barley can be used in soup or as a side dish. (Whole grain barley is more nutritious than pearl barley.) Bulgur, too, is a fine substitute for rice or potatoes. Get to know buckwheat and millet—both can be used as nutritious side dishes.

Sun exposure

The ultraviolet rays in sunlight cause skin cancer. This effect has been known since 1894, but skin cancer was rare in those days because a suntan wasn't fashionable. Skin cancer rates began rising in the 1930s, when clothing and bathing suits became more revealing and having a tan meant you had the money and the leisure time to spend hours in the sun. Today, malignant melanoma, the deadliest form of skin cancer, is the fastest-rising cancer in the United States, after lung cancer in women.

The three forms of skin cancer are linked to excessive sun exposure. They're most common in tropical and subtropical climates, and on areas of the body that go uncovered in warm weather. Like any other carcinogen, ultraviolet light causes cancer by damaging DNA. Your risk of malignant melanoma is especially high if you received a particularly severe sunburn as a child; basal and squamous cell carcinoma are associated with ultraviolet light damage that's been built up through years of sunning. Your risk is also high if you're fair-skinned and have light-colored hair and eyes. In general, the darker your natural coloring, the better protected you are against the carcinogenic effects of the sun. Ideally, the people at highest risk should wear a sunscreen every day.

The rays of the sun
Remember that the sun's rays are strong enough to tan or burn you even on cloudy, foggy, hazy days. Sand, water, and cement reflect the sun's rays. Even under a beach umbrella you're only protected from about 50 percent of the dangerous rays.

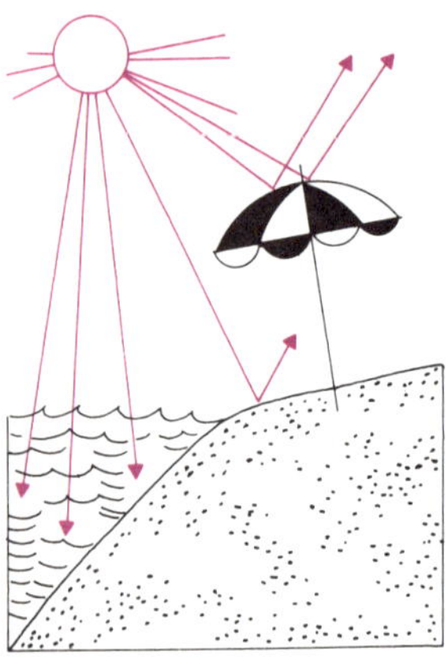

The dangers of too much sun are fairly well-known, but this knowledge hasn't stopped people from pursuing those golden tans that we ironically associate with good health. If the lily-white look just isn't for you, you can diminish the hazards of ultraviolet exposure by taking a few precautions.

1. Tan gradually. A slowly acquired tan will help build up melanin, a protective pigment that forms in your skin. If you burn before you've built up this protection, ultraviolet rays can penetrate to the skin's lower layers, where they do their damage.

2. Protect yourself when outdoors by using sunscreens—creams, lotions, and makeup that screen out the sun's harmful rays. A wide variety of these products is available, and they've been rated by their SPF (Sun Protection Factor). The SPF ranges from 2 to 15 according to the degree to which the product blocks

Skin types and recommended SPF

This chart matches skin types to recommended SPF ratings. Find your skin type in the column at left and read across to find the recommended SPF.

Skin type	Recommended SPF
Burns easily; never tans	8 or higher
Burns easily; tans minimally	6 to 7
Burns moderately; tans gradually	4 to 5
Rarely burns; always tans well	2 to 3
Rarely burns; tans easily	2

Avoid exposure during the most dangerous hours—when the sun is directly overhead. This is usually between 10 A.M. and 2 P.M. Early morning (before 10) and late afternoon (after 4) are the safest times of the day for enjoying the beach, pool, or outdoor activities.

out the sun's radiation. The higher the SPF, the more effective the product is in preventing sunburn.

Apply sunscreens liberally, and be sure to apply such products every few hours and after swimming. Put sunscreens on all exposed areas of skin, including the backs of your hands and even the tops of your ears. Make sure the product contains PABA (para-aminobenzoic acid), which blocks the sun's ultraviolet rays.

3. Remember that the sun's rays are strong enough to tan or burn you even on cloudy, foggy, hazy days. Sand, water, and cement (such as that around swimming pools) reflect the sun's rays. Even under a beach umbrella, you're only protected from about 50 percent of the dangerous rays. And staying in the water won't protect you either, because ultraviolet light passes through water.

4. You also risk sunburn when skiing or mountain climbing because snow reflects sunlight, which is more intense at higher altitudes. The sun's burning rays increase 4 percent in intensity for every 1,000 feet above sea level. If you like to spend your summers hiking at altitudes of 10,000 feet or more, you'll experience sunlight that's nearly half again as strong as that felt by your friends on the beach. You might want to adjust your SPF upward to compensate for this stronger ultraviolet exposure.

Malignant melanoma is almost 100 percent curable if detected in time. If allowed to progress, it spreads to the brain, bones, liver, and lungs, and ultimately kills. Check yourself regularly for this and other forms of skin cancer. In Chapter 3 (see pages 48 to 49), you'll learn how to do a complete skin self-examination, but two general warning signals you should look for are an ulcer or sore that doesn't heal, and any change in appearance of a wart or mole. These could indicate the presence of any of the three skin cancers. Remember, skin cancers are easily cured if caught early, but the chances of scarring and even death increase the longer you wait to get help.

Radiation

Radiation has been a recognized carcinogen since X-rays were discovered a century ago. Early radiologists, unprotected while they worked with X-rays, soon developed higher-than-expected rates of skin cancer and leukemia.

We're always exposed to small amounts of natural "background" radiation, such as that from sunlight or from natural radioactive substances in rocks and soil. The problem arises when this exposure becomes excessive. For example, we've seen that too much time in the sun places you at much higher risk for skin cancer. Survivors of the atomic blasts in Hiroshima and Nagasaki are now suffering from high rates of leukemia. Lung cancer also has been associated with too much radiation exposure.

How can you minimize your risks?

- *Minimize tanning and sunburn.*
- *Avoid unnecessary X-rays.*
- *When you must have X-rays, make sure your doctor or dentist takes all the proper precautions, like covering uninvolved parts of the body with lead shields or aprons.*

Pollutants and workplace carcinogens

The link between working conditions and cancer in humans is another source of debate. Since some cancers take a long time to develop, sometimes as long as 40 years, the controversy usually centers on cause and effect relationships. In the asbestos industry, for example, workers may show no cancer until 20 or 30 years after exposure to the fibers. For over 30 years, then, in-

Workplace hazards

Workers in many fields are exposed to substances that may cause cancer. This chart matches occupations with the suspected causes of cancer.

Occupation	Suspected cause of cancer
Automobile mechanic	Petroleum products
Carpenter	Wood dusts
Dyer	Aromatic amines, benzene
Leather worker	Leather dusts
Miner	Arsenic, asbestos, coal
Painter	Benzene
Potter	Chromium
Rubber worker	Aromatic amines, vinyl chloride
Shoemaker	Benzene
Textile printer	Cadmium
Welder	Cadmium

Smokers and industrial chemicals
Cigarette smokers who work with dangerous chemicals increase their risk of lung disease. The combined effects of cigarette smoke and exposure to industrial substances—such as fumes and dusts—make many workers especially susceptible to lung ailments. For example, smokers exposed to asbestos have a cancer risk nearly 60 times that of other people.

dustry leaders argued that asbestos dust was harmless and those who developed cancers had to try to establish that asbestos was the cause. At present, so-called workplace carcinogens contribute to about 4 percent of our yearly new cases.

Occupational cancers
Job-related cancers are often difficult to identify because they usually occur a decade or more after exposure, and that exposure may have been brief—sometimes only a few months. People may even forget they've been exposed at all, until the information is ferreted out by an astute doctor who asks the right questions.

The first person to recognize and describe an occupation-related cancer was the 18th-century English doctor Sir Percivall Pott, who noted the relationship between scrotal cancer in young chimney sweeps and their constant exposure to the dust and ashes in the chimneys. Since then, many other industrial carcinogens have been identified, usually through the painful experience of those unlucky enough to have worked with them. Examples of these include asbestos, radium, arsenic, and vinyl chloride monomer, a component of polyvinyl chloride, which is used in making plastic. Today, strict rules govern the use of workplace carcinogens, but several million workers are exposed nonetheless. For example, 2 to 3 million people work closely with a carcinogen called benzene, which is used in coke, rubber, and petrochemical plants, as well as in making artificial leather and rubber cement for shoes. Thus, shoemakers may be exposed to it as much as factory workers, gas station attendants, and furniture finishers. Similar situations exist with other chemicals.

What if you get one of these symptoms?
No symptom listed here necessarily means that you've got cancer. But you'll want to find out what is causing the symptom. See your doctor. Then what? If the symptom is that of a minor ailment, your doctor will take care of it. If the symptom uncovers cancer, you'll have the advantage of early detection, which means a much greater probability of cure.

Does this mean that those workers will inevitably develop cancer at some later date? Not necessarily. Hazards can be reduced when proper precautions are followed. Typical precautions include:

• controlled ventilation of a plant's air to remove dangerous vapors

• changes in work practices, such as allowing brief work periods for those exposed

• protective equipment, such as respirators, goggles, and nonabsorbent clothing

• regular, detailed checkups to maintain health and monitor physical changes.

The precautions aren't always followed, unfortunately. Managers in many smaller factories may not have the resources or the knowledge to protect their workers adequately. Larger companies may feel that a larger profit justifies keeping their workers uninformed as long as possible. While this statement may seem outrageous, asbestos manufacturers did, in fact, participate in an industry-wide cover-up that lasted for decades and destroyed the lives of thousands of people. Could the same thing occur today in other industries? Perhaps.

Workers need to inform themselves of any possible dangers associated with the material they're using and to scrupulously follow whatever safety guidelines are provided. If you're genuinely concerned about possible hazards in your workplace, alert your coworkers and superiors.

Understanding the risk factors

By knowing which factors place you in a high-risk category for cancer, you can be alert to any warning signals that occur and see your doctor for the earliest possible detection. This chart summarizes the major risk factors, as well as actions you can take to lower those risks.

Risk factor	Risk	Action
Cigarettes, cigars, pipes 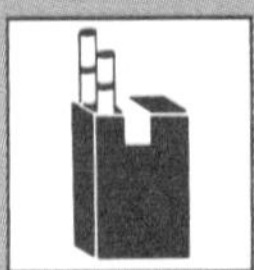	Increased risk of lung cancer.	Don't smoke.
Snuff, chewing tobacco 	Increased risk of oral cancer.	Don't use smokeless tobacco products.
Long-term use of high-dose estrogens 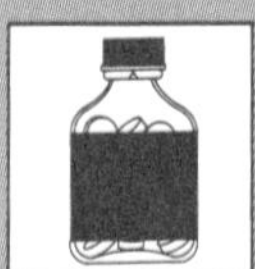	Increased risk of uterine cancer.	Avoid taking estrogens. If you must take them, use the smallest possible dose, for no longer than necessary. Discuss risks and benefits with your doctor.
Occupation 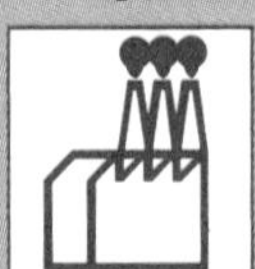	Exposure to one or a combination of certain known cancer-causing industrial agents (nickel, chromate, uranium, asbestos, petroleum, vinyl chloride), in many cases combined with smoking, leads to an increased risk of several cancers.	Industries can take a number of steps to reduce or eliminate occupational hazards. Become informed about the health and safety rules for your workplace. Don't smoke.

Risk factor	Risk	Action
Overexposure to X-rays (for example, a large number of X-rays over a long period of time) 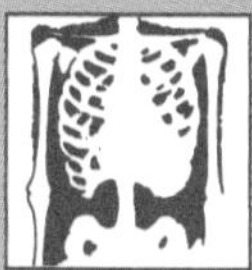	Increased risk of many types of cancers.	Avoid unnecessary X-rays. Be sure that X-ray shields are used to protect other parts of your body.
Sunlight 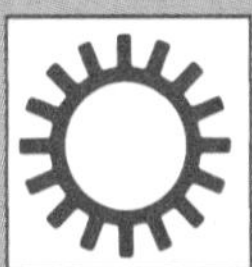	Long or repeated exposure with no sunscreen protection leads to increased risk of skin cancer.	Don't stay in the sun for more than brief periods without protection: hats, long sleeves, long pants, sunscreen lotions.
Heavy alcohol consumption 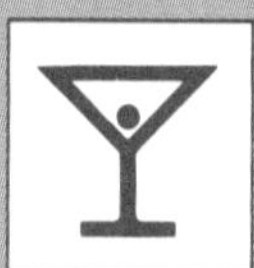	Increased risk of mouth, throat, liver, and esophageal cancer. Risk is multiplied when combined with cigarette smoking.	If you drink alcohol, do so only in moderation.
Diet high in fat and calories, low in fresh fruits, vegetables, grains 	Increased risk of several cancers.	Vary diet to include foods low in fat (fresh fruits, vegetables, whole-grain breads and cereals, low-fat dairy products, lean meat, poultry without the skin, fish, peas, beans). Prepare foods by baking, broiling, poaching, and simmering with little or no added fat, rather than frying. Use margarine, butter, oils, and salad dressings sparingly. Treat yourself to baked goods and desserts only on special occasions.

3 Early cancer detection

You can protect yourself
You'll be surprised at how many actions you can take to detect early cancers—the ones easiest to cure. If you use the warning signs and self-examination procedures in this chapter, you'll know about the health of those body areas that are most susceptible to cancers. Remember that knowing about your health is the key to keeping it.

Cancer's seven warning symptoms
The American Cancer Society stresses the importance of these seven warning symptoms. See your doctor if you experience any of these symptoms:
1. ***C**hange in bowel or bladder habits.*
2. ***A** sore that doesn't heal.*
3. ***U**nusual bleeding or discharge.*
4. ***T**hickening or lump in breast or elsewhere.*
5. ***I**ndigestion or difficulty in swallowing.*
6. ***O**bvious change in wart or mole.*
7. ***N**agging cough or hoarseness.*

The earlier a cancer is detected, the better the chances of its being cured. Treatment for a cancer caught in its earlier stages is much less radical and has fewer side effects than the treatments employed for more advanced cancer. Furthermore, the treatment for a cancer caught in its earlier stages may not require major disfiguring surgery. After prevention, then, early detection is the best approach. To take one example, with early treatment, the cure rate for cancer of the larynx is about 80 percent—that's 4 out of every 5 people who are treated for it in its early stages. Later detection and treatment yield only about a 25 percent cure rate—about 1 out of every 4 patients.

The American Cancer Society has identified seven basic warning symptoms that everyone should know. (Other specific warning symptoms are associated with specific cancers.) Most of these symptoms can be spotted by doing self-examination of the area involved. Self-examination means you can examine the area yourself, without a doctor's help and without special equipment. With self-examination, you'll greatly improve the probability of detecting any cancer while it's still at a highly curable stage. Learning how to examine your body can save your life. This is especially true of breast self-examination in women.

Now for a word of caution: cancer symptoms can indicate a problem other than cancer. Don't ever leap to the conclusion that you have cancer based solely on an examination you've done on yourself at home. Lumps, bumps, and similar changes are reflections of any number of conditions; the odds that they're cancer are quite small. So don't panic if one or more of these symptoms turn up on you; just see your doctor as soon as you can. And remember: even if it does turn out to be cancer, prompt diagnosis and treatment lead to a cure much of the time.

General warning symptoms

According to the American Cancer Society, the most obvious cancer warning symptoms are:

• Change in bowel or bladder habits. This could indicate cancer of the bladder, colon, rectum, or prostate. Bowel changes, which include constipation or diarrhea, rectal bleeding, and gas pains that get worse as the cancer grows, are often the result of an obstruction caused by a tumor in the area. Bladder changes include difficult, painful, or bloody urination, and may signal cancer of either the bladder or prostate.

Are you risking cancer?

How do you know if you're at high risk for cancer? You are if you have any of the following characteristics:

- *You drink heavily or smoke.*
- *Certain forms of cancer run in your family.*
- *You spend (or have spent) a lot of time in the sun.*
- *You're 40 percent or greater overweight and get 40 percent or more of your daily calories from fats.*
- *You've been exposed to a lot of radiation or certain occupational hazards.*

• A sore that doesn't heal. This could be a forerunner of skin cancer or, if it appears in the mouth, of mouth cancer. If you see or feel a sore, a lump, a thickening, or a raised, irregular, or warty area on your cheek, gum, or tongue, show it to your doctor or dentist. The self-examination of your mouth is described in more detail on page 49.

• Unusual bleeding or discharge. This may indicate cancer of the colon or womb (uterus). Blood in the stool is an important warning symptom of colon cancer, but it's also common in people with bleeding hemorrhoids or diseases like colitis. Unusual vaginal bleeding, such as after intercourse, between periods, or after menopause, may signal early uterine or late cervical cancer. When caught early enough, these forms of cancer are usually cured. A Pap smear, a test performed by a doctor, can detect cervical cancer long before it manifests itself as abnormal bleeding. It's described on pages 41 and 46.

• Thickening or lump in the breast or elsewhere. The majority of breast lumps aren't cancer, but if you find one during a breast self-examination, visit your doctor immediately. Of those who receive early treatment, 85 percent of women with breast cancer are alive and show no disease after 5 years—the official definition of a cancer cure. Early discovery and prompt treatment of breast cancer saves lives. Lumps elsewhere, such as on the neck or groin, occasionally indicate the presence of cancer in the lymph nodes in those areas and require immediate medical attention.

• Indigestion or difficulty swallowing. Tumors in the stomach or esophagus may produce these symptoms. Symptoms of indigestion, such as mild pain or discomfort, feeling full or bloated, slight nausea, heartburn, loss of appetite, belching, or vomiting, are the most common symptoms of stomach cancer. Difficulty in swallowing may be due to a tumor that obstructs the esophagus.

Don't be alarmed if you have one of these symptoms. By itself, it may indicate nothing more than a minor ailment of the digestive tract, but see your doctor.

• Obvious change in a wart or mole. This early symptom of skin cancer may take the form of a dry, scaly patch; a persistent pimple; an inflamed area with a crusty center; or a pale, waxy, or pearly nodule that may eventually ulcerate.

Malignant melanoma may first appear as a small, dark, molelike growth that enlarges, ulcerates, or bleeds. It sometimes arises in a mole that you've always had.

• Nagging cough or hoarseness. A persistent cough is sometimes, but not always, a symptom of lung cancer. Cancer in the bronchi, or air passages of the lung, may obstruct or irritate the passages, leading to a cough and sometimes making the patient cough up blood. Cancer in other parts of the lung may cause no symptoms at all and may be detected only at a very late stage, by X-ray. As of now, no one knows a reliable test for the early detection of lung cancer.

Nagging hoarseness may be a symptom of cancer of the larynx. Sometimes the symptoms are mild and may be attributed to a cold, too much smoking, or an unusual amount of talking. Have your doctor check your hoarseness, though; it's an early symptom, and treatment carries a good chance of cure with little effect on the voice.

Other warning symptoms

• Vomiting blood. It may be red or it may be darker and resemble coffee grounds.

• Persistent pain. Pain anywhere lasting more than a few days is a sign that something is wrong and should be investigated.

• Anemia. Anemia, especially in women past menopause, often indicates internal bleeding, usually from the stomach or intestine. This isn't necessarily an indication of cancer, but bleeding is always serious.

Here again, these general symptoms may indicate many other things besides cancer. Put your mind at ease by promptly having a thorough checkup. Even when not caused by a tumor, none of these problems should be allowed to go untreated.

Breast self-examination

Women find up to 90 percent of all cases of breast cancer during their breast self-examination. If you're female and age 20 or older, examine yourself once a month using these simple ways: while taking a shower or while standing in front of a mirror, and while lying down. If you're not sure you're examining yourself thoroughly, ask your doctor or nurse to teach you.

For women

Mammograms and Pap smears must be done by a doctor. Both are painless, essential examinations. Mammograms can detect breast tumors too small for you to feel, and you should have one after your 35th birthday. Pap smears confirm the health of cervix cells. You should have your first Pap test when you're 20 years old.

Mammography

A mammogram is a low-dose breast X-ray that's first done in women who are age 35 or older. Mammography can detect cancers too small to be felt by hand; the American Cancer Society considers this and the breast self-examination the two best ways of detecting breast cancer. The society makes these recommendations:

- A woman age 20 or older should do a monthly breast self-examination and receive a professional breast examination by her doctor or nurse every 3 years until age 40.
- Between the ages of 35 and 40, a woman should have her first mammogram. Called a "baseline" mammogram, it provides a picture of her breasts under normal conditions and offers a basis of comparison for future tests. She should continue the monthly breast self-examination and get a professional breast checkup every 3 years.
- Between the ages of 40 and 49, a woman should receive a mammogram every 1 to 2 years, as well as continue her breast examinations monthly and have her annual checkup.
- Once she reaches age 50, a woman should have a mammogram yearly, while she continues to examine her breasts monthly and have an annual checkup.

The Pap smear

Named for Dr. George N. Papanicolaou, who developed the test in the 1920s, the Pap smear (or test) is a fast, painless, and inexpensive method of detecting cervical cancer at a stage when it's still 100 percent curable. Thanks largely to this test, deaths from cervical cancer have declined dramatically.

The test, which can be done by a doctor during a routine gynecological examination, consists of collecting cells from the cervix and vagina with a stick or a cotton swab. The cells are smeared onto a glass slide and examined under a microscope. A Pap test's results are called "normal" or "abnormal" rather than "posi-

(text continued on page 46)

Breast self-examination

You should perform these self-examinations once a month, at the same time.

In the shower

You can easily examine your breasts during a bath or shower because your hands will glide more easily over wet skin. To examine your right breast, raise your arm behind your head; keeping the fingers of your left hand flat, gently press the entire breast. Reverse this procedure for your left breast. Check for any lump, hardening, or thickening.

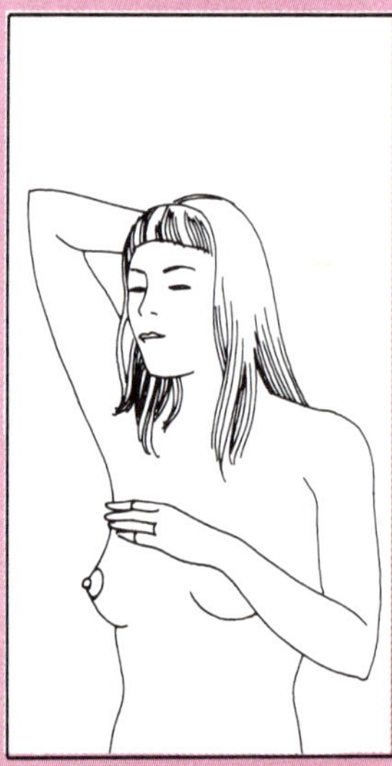

In front of a mirror

First look at your breasts with your arms hanging at your sides.

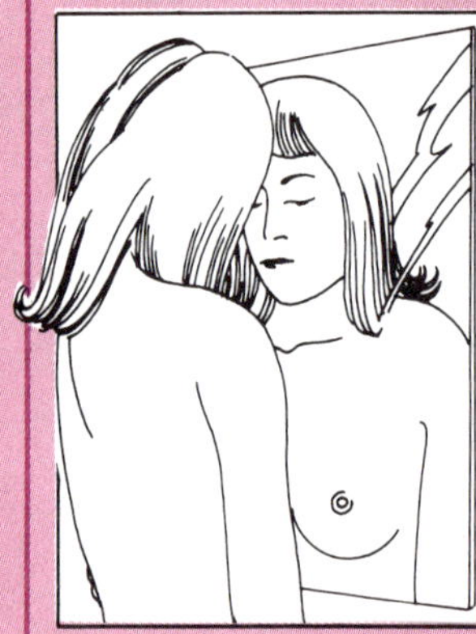

Then raise your arms. Check for any changes in the shape of each breast, a swelling, dimpling of the skin, or changes in the nipples.

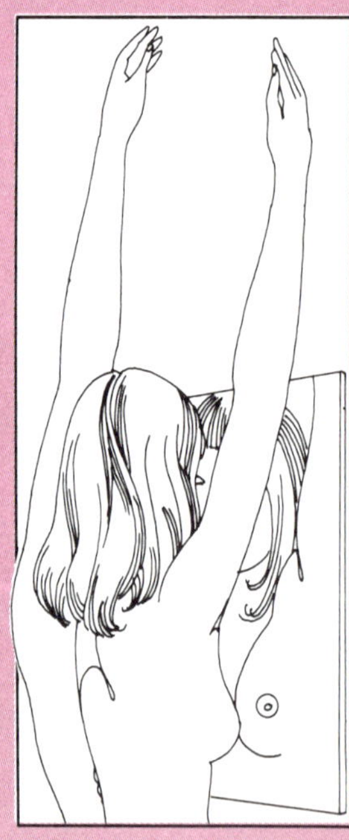

Then rest your hands on your hips and press down firmly, flexing your chest muscles. Don't expect both breasts to look exactly the same—few women's breasts do. Once you do this examination a few months in a row, you'll learn what looks normal for you, and you'll more easily spot any changes that might occur.

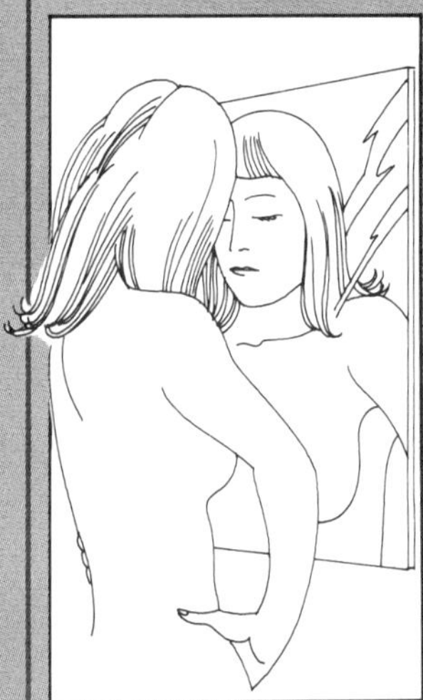

On your back

To examine your right breast, put a pillow or a folded towel under your right shoulder. To distribute the breast tissue more evenly on the chest, put your right hand behind your head.

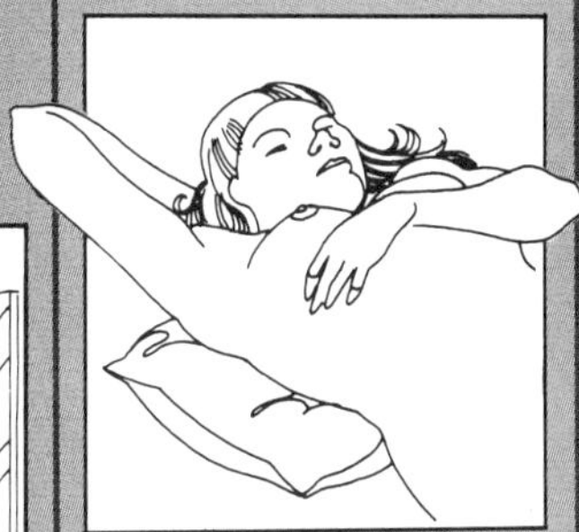

Using your left hand, fingers flat, press gently around your right breast in small, clockwise, circular motions, as though you were feeling the face of a clock. Think of the top, outermost portion of your right breast as 12 o'clock, then move to 1 o'clock, and so on, until you've completed the circle and are back at 12. Don't be alarmed if you find a ridge of firm tissue in the lower curve of the breast: this is normal.

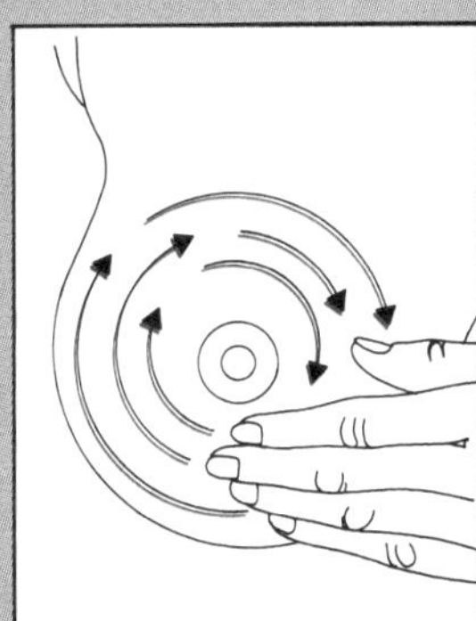

Repeat the circle by moving your hand about an inch closer to your nipple and starting again. You should examine every part of your breast, each time moving your hand a little closer to the nipple. Repeat this process and examine your left breast with your right hand.

One final check

Finally, squeeze the nipple of each breast gently between your thumb and index finger. Any discharge, clear or bloody, should be reported to your doctor immediately.

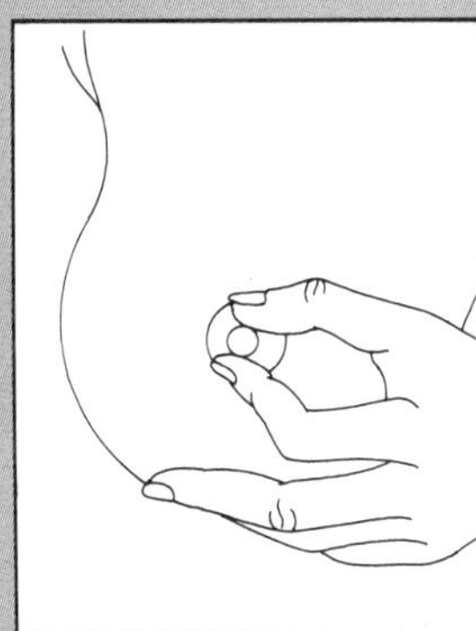

Changing patterns for major cancers

These graphs show the changes that have taken place in the death rates for adult men and women from eight major cancers: lung, breast, colon and rectum,

Lung

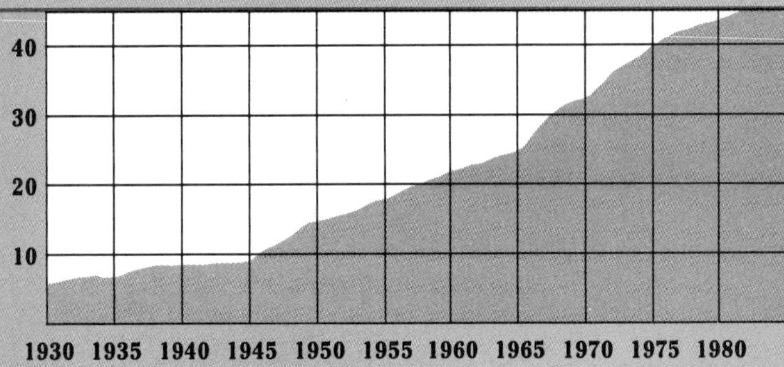

Breast

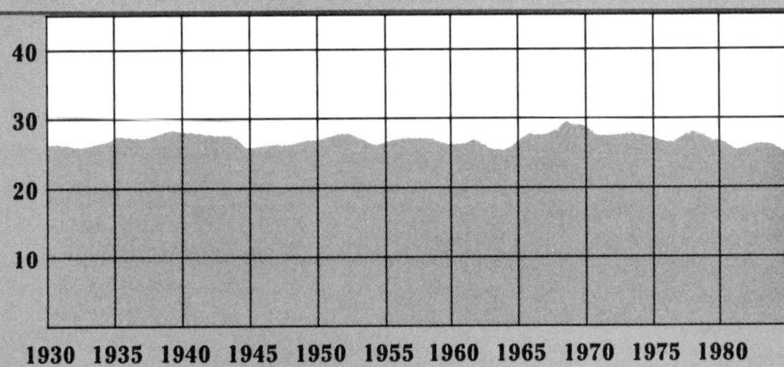

Colon and rectum

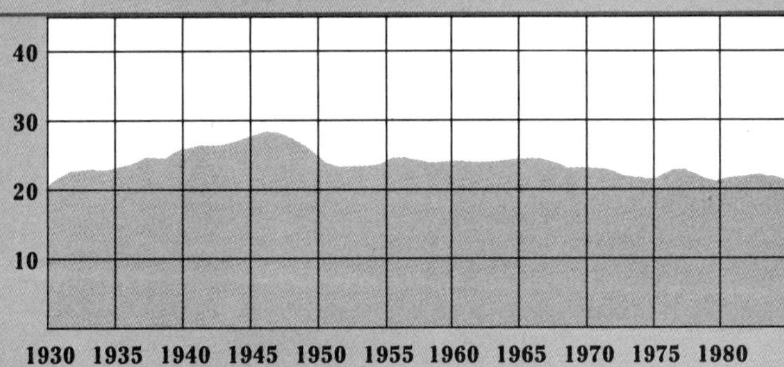

Prostate

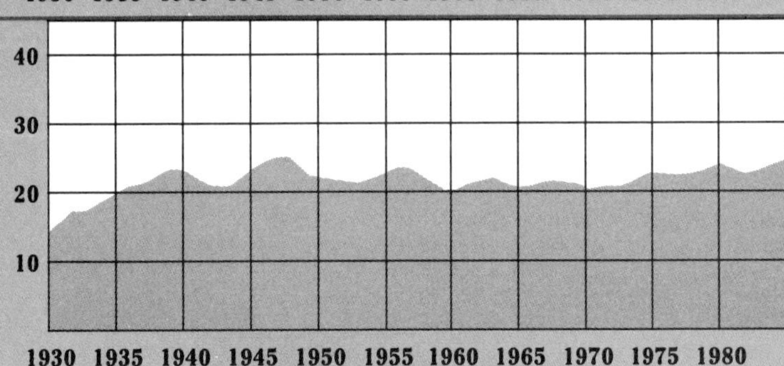

prostate, uterus, stomach, leukemia, and pancreas. These approximate figures are given as the percentage per 100,000 people in the United States.

Uterus

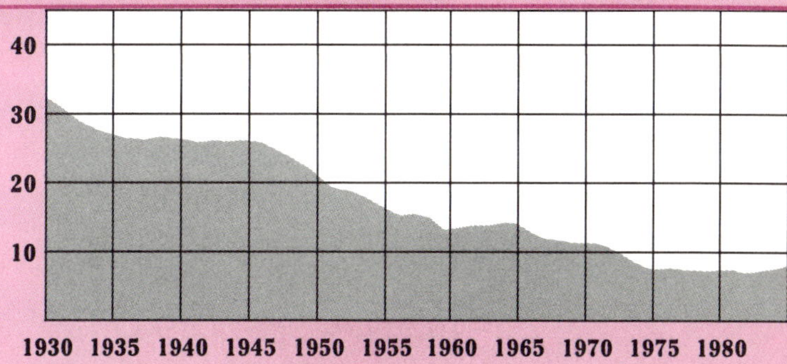

Stomach

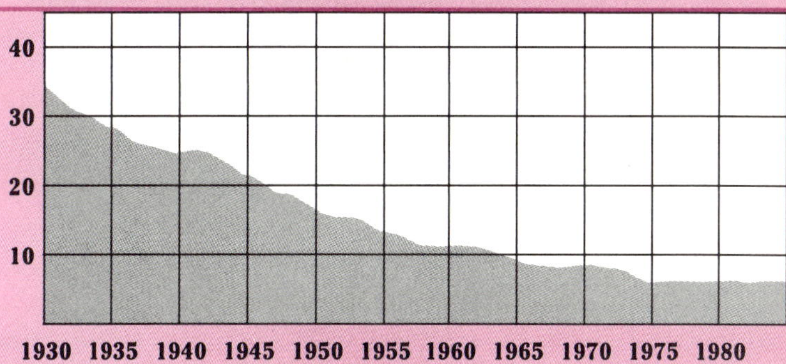

Blood (Leukemia)

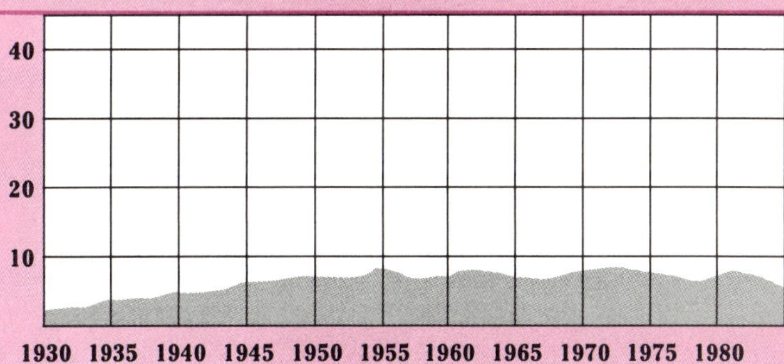

Pancreas

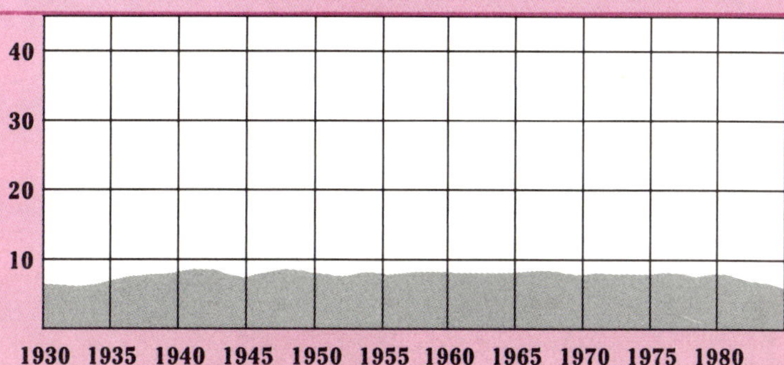

tive" or "negative." An abnormal Pap smear is found in about 1 out of every 20 women, and it's *not* a definitive diagnosis of cancer. It means an abnormality that must be investigated is present. An abnormal Pap smear may be caused by an infection, which is usually treated with antibiotics, or by a condition called dysplasia. Dysplasia is a change in cervical cells that leads to cancer in about one-third of all cases. It goes away on its own in another third, and stays the same in the final third. However, all cases must be treated immediately, because doctors have no way of knowing which cases will become more severe. Dysplasia has no symptoms, so only a Pap smear can detect it. Depending on its severity, and the woman's needs (for example, her age and her desire to have children), treatment for cervical dysplasia may range from a simple freezing procedure that destroys abnormal cells, to surgery.

The American Cancer Society recommends that when a woman reaches age 20 she have a Pap smear and another one the following year. If the two tests are normal, she should have one every 3 years after that.

The prostate
As the prostate gland expands, it compresses the urethra and bladder, obstructing urine flow. The prostate enlarges to a certain degree with age, but it can also become a tumor, so consult your doctor when you suspect prostate problems.

Prostate cancer

Prostate cancer strikes about 18 percent of American men, mostly after age 55. In the past, this was often a traumatic experience for a man because treatment almost always left him impotent. New treatments now preserve potency in the great majority of cases detected early. Thus, heed the early warning symptoms:

- Weak or interrupted urine flow.
- The need to urinate frequently, especially at night.

Normal prostate

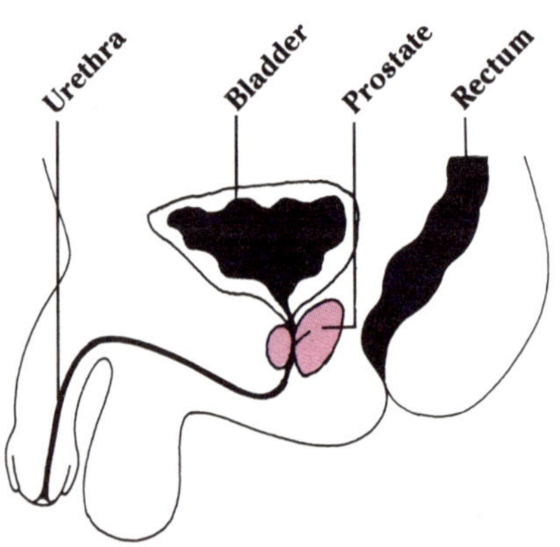

Enlarged prostate

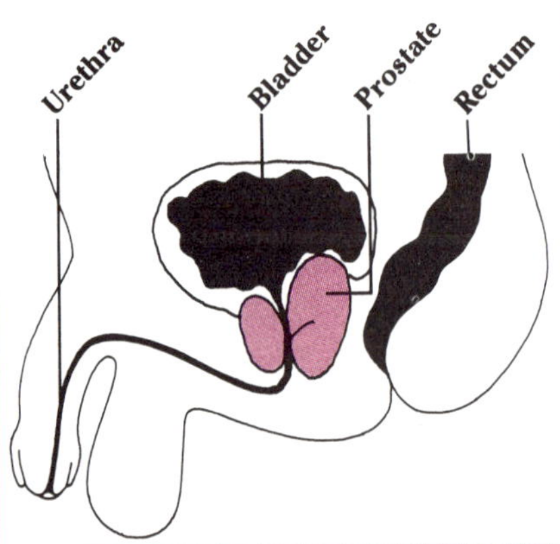

- Inability to urinate or trouble starting to urinate under usual conditions.
- Blood in the urine.
- Pain or burning during urination.
- Constant pain in the lower back, pelvis, or thighs.

Reasons unknown
For reasons that no one understands, testicular cancer concentrates in men aged 20 to 34. Therefore, every male between 20 and 34 should give himself a monthly testicular self-examination.

The best way to detect prostate cancer early is through a rectal examination, which should be part of an annual checkup for every man after age 40.

Testicular self-examination
Testicular cancer is very rare, striking less than 1 percent of American men. However, it's one of the most common cancers in men between the ages of 20 and 34. (Most cancers strike people older than 65.) Testicular cancer accounts for 22 percent of the cancer deaths in young white men. No one knows what causes it, but it's characterized by tumors that most often develop in the right rather than the left testicle, often in an undescended testicle.

Fortunately, if caught in time, testicular cancer is almost 100 percent curable and has no effect on a man's potency. A man should give himself a monthly testicular self-examination for tumors, right after a hot bath or shower. Most cases of testicular cancer are caught by the men themselves.

Testicular self-examination

Here's how to do your testicular self-examination:

While standing or lying down, gently examine each testicle with the fingers of both hands: thumbs on top, middle and index fingers on the bottom. Roll the testicle between your fingers, making sure you feel the entire area of each testicle. Feel for size, shape, consistency, and sensitivity to pressure. After you've done this for a few months, you'll get to know what's normal for you: as with women's breasts, men's testicles are never completely symmetrical. A firm, painless swelling of one testicle may indicate cancer. Here again, however, it could also indicate many other things: see your doctor.

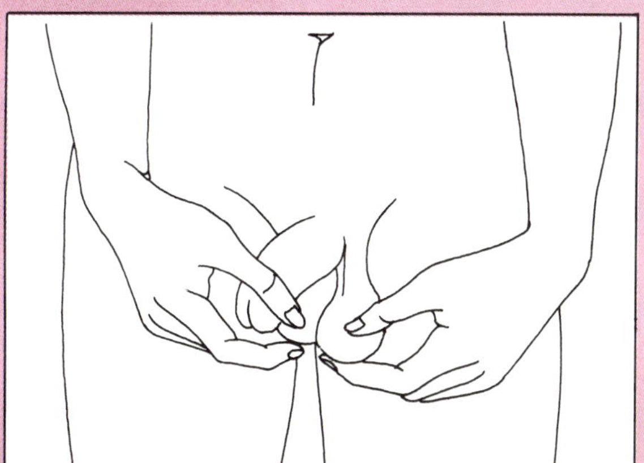

Lumps, moles, and other skin changes: early detection of skin cancer

Early detection and treatment of skin cancer virtually guarantee its cure. As with the other forms of cancer mentioned in this chapter, a suspicious-looking change in the skin isn't difficult to spot, once you get to know your body and what's normal for it.

You should give yourself a thorough skin self-examination at least once a year. As one dermatologist suggests, "Examine your birthday suit on your birthday." To distinguish early malignant melanoma from a normal mole or freckle, remember the ABCD rule: *A*symmetry, *B*order, *C*olor, and *D*iameter.

- Asymmetry. A malignant melanoma is asymmetrical. That is, if you drew a line down its center, the two halves wouldn't match. Normal skin markings are usually more symmetrical.
- Border. The borders of a malignant melanoma are often notched or uneven, while those of normal moles or freckles are usually even or smooth.
- Color. A malignant melanoma may contain mixed shades of several colors, unlike a normal mark, which is usually all one color.
- Diameter. A malignant melanoma is usually wider than a pencil eraser, making it larger than most normal freckles and moles.

Since melanoma is the deadliest of the skin cancers, learn its warning symptoms.

Other skin changes may indicate basal or squamous cell carcinomas. An early basal cell carcinoma may appear as a lump with one or more of the following characteristics:

- Smooth, round, waxy appearance.
- Raised, sometimes pearly edges.
- A surface crisscrossed with enlarged blood vessels.
- Intermittent bleeding and crusting over: the lump may disappear temporarily, but never really heals.
- Up to 1 inch in diameter.

Squamous cell carcinomas are often preceded by what dermatologists call a premalignant change. The most common of these is called a solar, or actinic, keratosis—a pink, white, yellow, or brown patch, most often found on wrinkled or weather-beaten skin. If you run your finger over it, it feels crusty or like little thorns. Prompt treatment greatly decreases the risk of

Changes in a mole

Watch for suspicious changes in your skin. Such changes may be early warning symptoms of cancer. Fortunately, spotting changes isn't difficult once you get to know your body and what's normal for it. Watch for these changes:

- *Asymmetry. Most skin cancers are asymmetrical. If you drew a line down the center of a cancerous growth, the two halves wouldn't match.*
- *Border. The borders of skin cancers are often notched or uneven, while those of normal moles or freckles are usually even or smooth.*
- *Color. A skin cancer may contain mixed shades of several colors, unlike a normal mark, which is usually all one color.*
- *Diameter. A skin cancer is usually wider than a pencil eraser, making it larger than most normal freckles or moles.*

Skin cancers are easy to cure. Indeed, early detection and treatment of skin cancer virtually guarantee its cure.

skin cancer in these areas, but if not treated, about 25 percent of the people with solar keratoses will develop squamous cell carcinoma. Treatment is easy: patients are usually given a prescription for a cream that they can apply at home several times a day for a few weeks.

Other possible characteristics of an early squamous cell carcinoma nodule include:

- a diameter of 1 inch or more
- a spot raised from the rest of the skin, with a pink color, an open center, and a hard border
- a spot on the lip that looks at first like a small eroded area.

Some general skin changes you should watch for include:

- any sore that doesn't heal or that heals and then reopens
- a thickening of any area of the skin
- a change in size or color of any mark that you've always had
- a persistent pain, itch, crusting, or bleeding of any spot.

Mouth self-examination

A thorough examination consists of the following steps: Feel your neck and cheeks for lumps or numb spots. Examine your face, neck, and lips in the mirror for any lumps, sores, or changes in color. If you wear glasses, remove them before doing this part of the exam, providing you can see well enough without them to detect any changes. While still in front of the mirror, and using a good light, open your mouth and examine its roof and floor for sores, lumps, or changes in color. Gently press the floor of your mouth with your finger to feel for lumps.

Examine your inner cheeks for any red, white, or darkened areas. Check your tongue for any lumps, swellings, or changes in color.

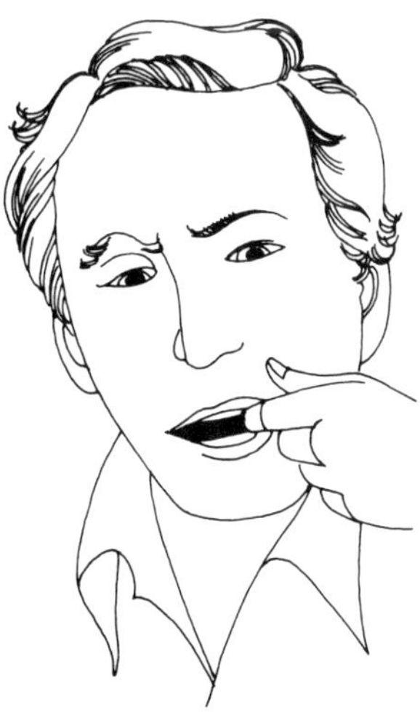

Early detection of mouth cancer: the mouth self-examination

Cancers of the mouth and throat appear twice as often in men as in women, especially after age 40 and in people who drink heavily and smoke. General warning symptoms of possible mouth cancer include:

- a sore in the mouth that bleeds easily and doesn't heal
- a lump or thickening in the mouth or on the neck
- a reddish or whitish patch that doesn't go away
- difficulty in chewing or swallowing food, or in moving the jaw or tongue.

The American Cancer Society recommends that you examine yourself for mouth cancer once a month.

You should also have an annual dental examination and ask your dentist to inspect your teeth, gums, tongue, and the floor of your mouth for possible signs of cancer.

Examining your lymph nodes

Axillary lymph nodes

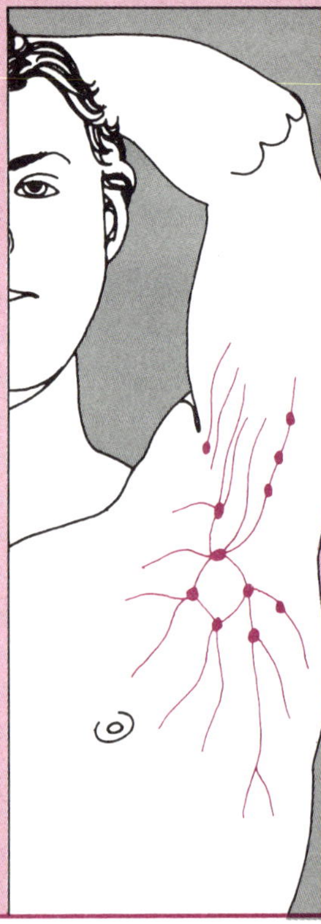

To do your armpit examination: with one arm hanging at your side, put the opposite hand in your armpit and press firmly but gently. Continue feeling down to the ribs on that side. You won't be able to feel all the lymph nodes, but those that you do feel should be no larger than beans.

Repeat the examination on the other side.

Lymph node self-examination

Lymph is the fluid that bathes and surrounds cells. Substances that are too large to be absorbed through the pores in the blood vessels enter the lymph, which eventually empties into the blood at a point near the heart. Because foreign invaders like germs or tumor cells are usually too large to enter the bloodstream, these substances reach the lymph. The lymph eventually travels to immune centers known as lymph nodes, where the body tries to destroy foreign or invading substances. Thus, when a tumor starts shedding cells, a nearby lymph node that is unable to destroy those cells could become another cancer site.

A lymph node is roughly the size and shape of a bean. When you do your self-examination, check for any swollen areas. This by itself isn't cause for panic, because lymph nodes often swell when your body is fighting off infections like a bad cold. Still, bring a swollen lymph node to your doctor's attention. Three im-

Neck lymph nodes

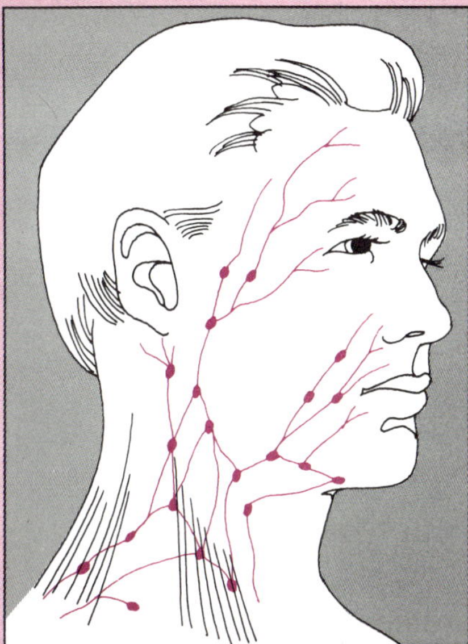

To do your neck examination, feel in front of and behind your ears, and at the base of your skull. Next, feel along the jawbone and chin. Press along the neck muscles under the ear, feeling all the way down to the collarbone.

Groin lymph nodes

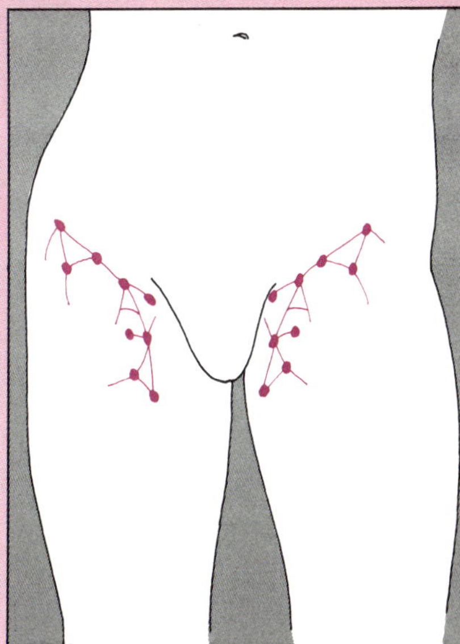

To do your self-examination, feel along your groin for any hard, painless swelling. Be sure to check both sides.

portant areas where you should do a lymph node self-examination are the neck, the axilla or armpit, and the groin.

Neck
Lymph nodes in the neck may be targets of spreading head and neck tumors.

Axilla
Axillary lymph nodes are frequent areas for the spread of breast cancer because they're very close to the breasts.

Groin
Swelling of lymph nodes in the groin is sometimes the first symptom of leukemia or of lymph node cancer, like Hodgkin's disease. To do your self-examination, feel along your groin for any hard, painless swelling. Be sure to check both sides. And remember, these nodes enlarge with infection, including a cold.

(text continued on page 56)

Cautionary steps to take

Most of the major forms of cancer have enough early warning symptoms for you to catch them while they're still highly curable. If you don't spot them during a self-examination, your doctor or

If you're age 20 to 40

Get a cancer-related checkup every 3 years. It should include the procedures listed below, plus health counseling (such as tips on quitting cigarettes) and examinations for cancer of the thyroid, testicles, prostate, mouth, ovaries, skin, and lymph nodes. Some people are at higher risk for certain cancers and may need to be tested more frequently.

Breast

An examination by a doctor every 3 years.
A self-examination every month.
One baseline mammogram between the ages of 35 and 40.

Uterus

A pelvic examination every 3 years.
A Pap test (after two initial normal tests one year apart) at least every 3 years, starting before age 20 in women who are sexually active.

Cancer in children
Cancers in children are often difficult to recognize because their symptoms may be taken for unimportant disorders. Children should have regular medical checkups, and parents should be alert to any unusual and persistent symptoms. Such symptoms include unusual lumps, double vision, nosebleeds, drowsiness, or listlessness.

dentist might during a routine examination. For people with no warning symptoms, the American Cancer Society makes the following suggestions.

If you're age 40 and above

Have a cancer-related checkup every year, including procedures listed below and health counseling and examinations for cancer of the thyroid, testicles, prostate, mouth, ovaries, skin, and lymph nodes. People at higher risks for certain cancers may need to be tested more frequently.

Breast

An examination by a doctor every year.
A self-examination every month.
A mammogram every year after age 50; between the ages of 40 and 50, ask your doctor.

Uterus

A pelvic examination every year.
A Pap test (after two initial normal tests one year apart) at least every 3 years.
An endometrial tissue sample taken by your doctor at menopause or if you're at risk (are infertile, obese, don't ovulate, have abnormal uterine bleeding, or are on estrogen therapy).

Colon and rectum

A rectal exam every year.
A Guaiac slide test (a test for blood in the stool) every year after age 50.
A proctological examination (after two initial negative tests one year apart) every 3 to 5 years after age 50.

Two kinds of cancer safeguards

Safeguards you do yourself

Lung

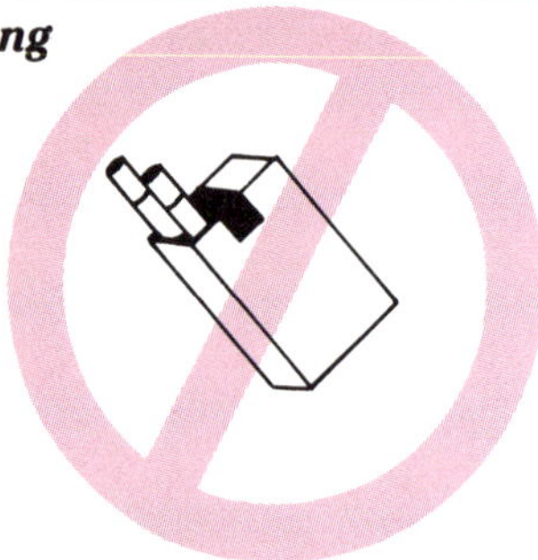

Don't smoke cigarettes
33 million Americans have quit. You can too.

Skin

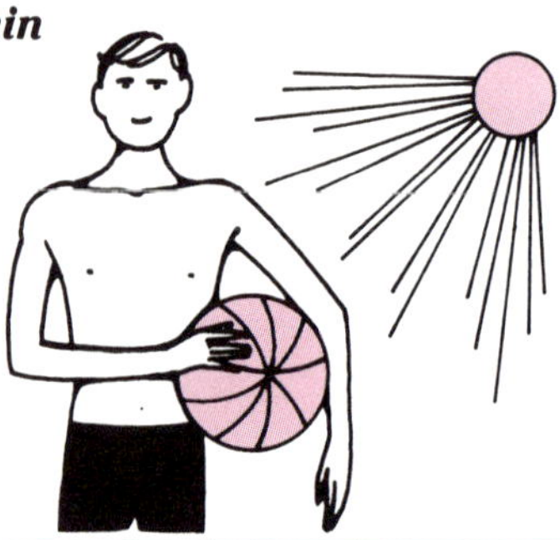

Avoid overexposure to the sun
Use sunscreens and protective clothing.

Breast

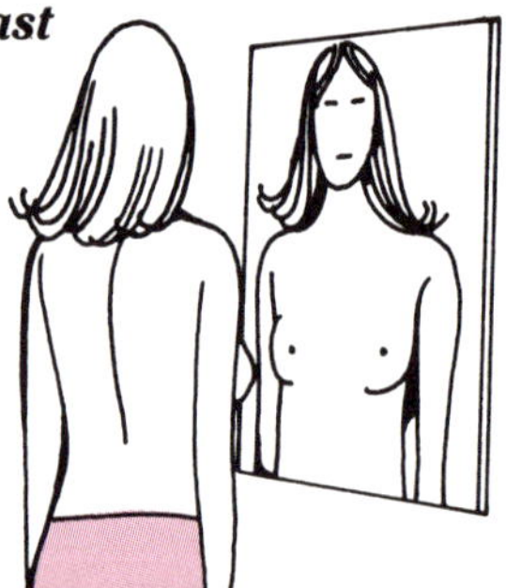

Monthly self-examination
Practice monthly breast self-examination, plus regular examinations by a physician.

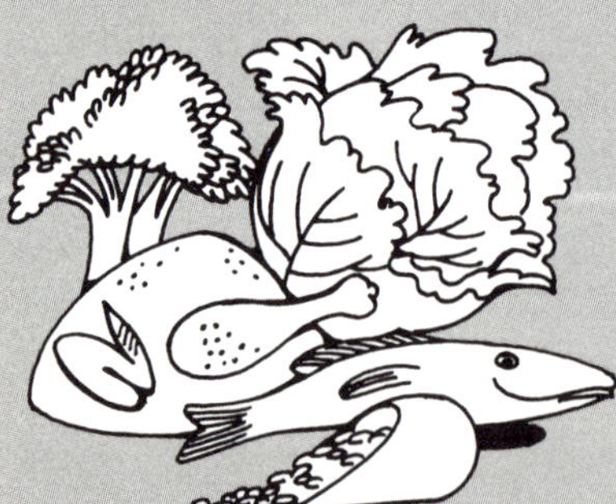

Eat an anticancer diet
Follow the tips provided in Chapter 2 for a healthy, anticancer diet.

Safeguards your doctor does

Mouth

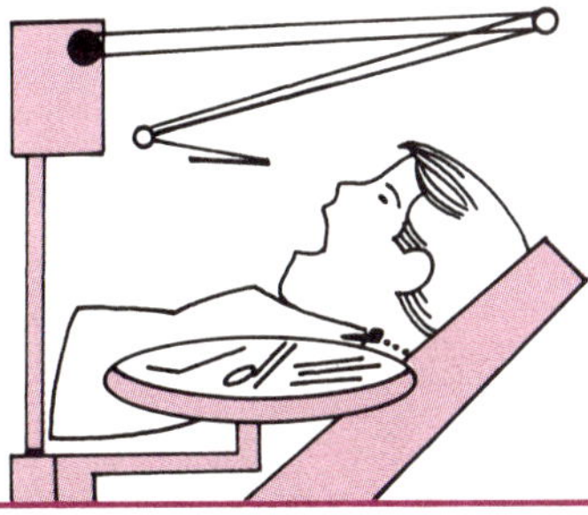

Regular examinations
Your physician or dentist can easily detect mouth cancer.

Uterus

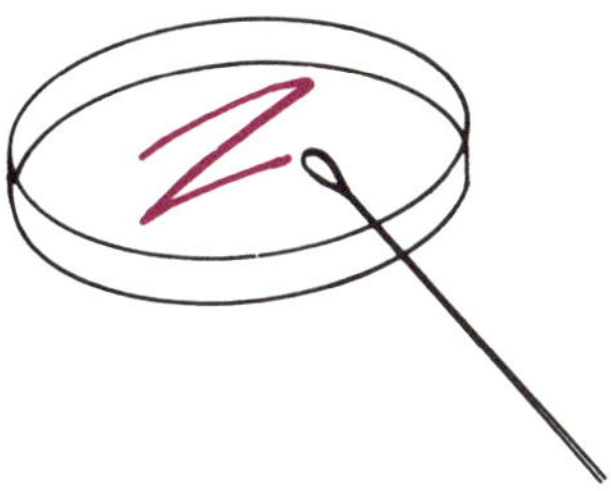

Pap test and pelvic examinations
If you are 20 or over (or younger and sexually active), have this test at least every 3 years, after two initial normal tests one year apart. A regular pelvic examination is also recommended.

Colon and rectum

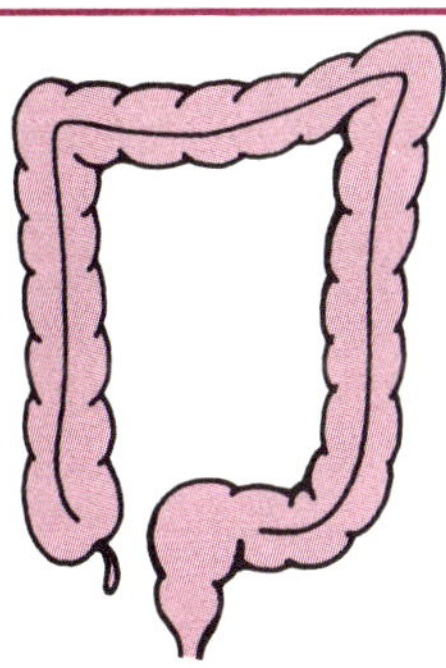

Colorectal cancer tests
After 40, have an annual digital rectal examination. After 50, include an annual stool occult blood test and a proctological examination after two initial negative tests one year apart.

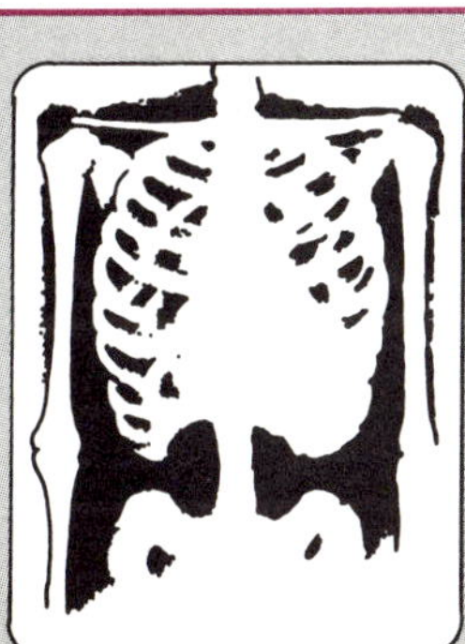

Cancer-related checkups
Have these checkups regularly. Ask your physician how often you should have one.

Some people are at higher risk for certain cancers and may need to have tests more frequently.

4 Confirming the diagnosis

What will happen next?

After you've had a warning symptom, you'll need tests that tell the possible causes. Follow-up tests may also be necessary. Then your doctor will work up an action plan for treating you. That may involve other doctors who are specialists for the cancer—if you have cancer.

Once you've spotted a cancer warning symptom and pointed it out to your doctor, he or she, after a preliminary examination, may want you to take more tests. This recommendation doesn't mean you actually have cancer—it means that your doctor needs more information for a definitive diagnosis.

Specialists use over 100 different tests for diagnosing cancers. The tests you take will depend on the suspected location of your cancer and whether or not doctors think it has spread. If your tests are extensive, remember that your doctors must know where a cancer is, how big it is, whether it has spread, and, if it has, where it has spread. The doctors must also know your medical history, something about your job and lifestyle, and your family's medical history as well. This information will help them make a thorough diagnosis and plan the most effective treatment for you.

The diagnostic process does little to dispel people's fears about cancer. Many tests are painful, embarrassing, and expensive; some require hospital stays and exposure to frightening-looking equipment. You'll probably be seen by numerous people: doctors, nurses, and technicians. Waiting for test results adds to the stress. This can be a harrowing time for the patient and for loved ones.

One thing you can do to alleviate the stress somewhat is to learn all you can about what's going on. Ask as many questions as necessary to prepare yourself for what's going to happen to you. You'll find some suggested questions below, but you should ask any question that will make the procedures more understandable. If you can't talk to the person who actually administers the tests, talk to your regular doctor—family physician, internist, gynecologist, or whomever you trust. He or she will remain your doctor throughout the testing process. If you do indeed have cancer, a cancer specialist will probably become your official doctor.

If you must have X-rays

If you've recently had X-rays taken by another doctor, ask if they can be used instead of new ones. If you're pregnant or may be pregnant, tell your doctor before an X-ray series. If you don't understand what the X-rays will tell your doctor, ask.

Don't be afraid to ask any questions about your tests.

Questions to ask

Good communication with your doctor is always important, but once you're suspected of having cancer, it becomes essential. You have a right to know what your tests will involve, how they'll feel, how much they'll cost, how long they'll take, and any other pertinent information. Discussing your fears and concerns with your doctor will serve two purposes: make you feel better and relax you. Relaxation is often necessary for the best test results.

Doctors and nurses who treat cancer patients—or potential cancer patients—know the terrible stress and fear these tests provoke. Don't be afraid of annoying them or taking up their time with questions.

Suggested general questions

Will I have any pain? (Hospital personnel often say "discomfort" when they mean "pain." Clarify this, as well as any other terms you don't understand.)

Will I need anesthesia for the test? Will I be put to sleep or will the doctor use a local painkiller? What are the side effects of the anesthesia?

Is this test dangerous to me? And what are the risks?

How long does the test take? Will I have to prepare for it in any special way?

If the test is painful, how severe will my pain be? How long will it last? Can you give me an example of what it will feel like?

What are the side effects from the tests themselves? How serious will they be, and how long will they last?

Will I need to stay in the hospital because of the test or the side effects it causes? If so, for how long?

How much will it cost? Is it covered by my insurance?

Making the diagnosis

If your doctors suspect you have cancer, they'll need as much basic information as you can give. This means they'll take an extensive medical history and do a thorough physical examination. The doctors will need such data as:

- your height and weight
- information on your breathing and heartbeat
- information about your eyes, ears, nose, and mouth
- the condition of the lymph nodes in your neck, groin, and armpits
- analyses of your blood, urine, and, if necessary, sputum and feces.

If they can get a tissue sample of the area in question without too much difficulty, as with a Pap smear, they'll do that, too.

Based on the results of these tests, your doctors may conclude that cancer isn't present, or they may need still more information and schedule you for more tests.

Looking inside
Tests designed to give doctors a view of your internal organs can be done in three general ways: through X-rays and scans, which involve the use of special films and contrast media; through ultrasound; and with surgery, which includes procedures like biopsies and endoscopies.

X-rays and scans

X-rays and scans often require the administration of a dye or contrast material, like barium, to enable doctors to view an internal organ more easily. Depending on the substance used and the organ involved, the material may be swallowed, injected, or given through an enema (inserted into the intestines by way of the anus).

To do a scan, a doctor will inject a radioactive substance into your body. Some forms of this substance are absorbed only by normal tissue, while other forms

What happens in a needle biopsy
In a biopsy, the doctor removes fluids and cells from an organ like a kidney or the liver. These samples can be studied and tested. The illustration at right shows a needle biopsy, in which the doctor inserts a needle into a tumor or growth and removes a small piece for analysis.

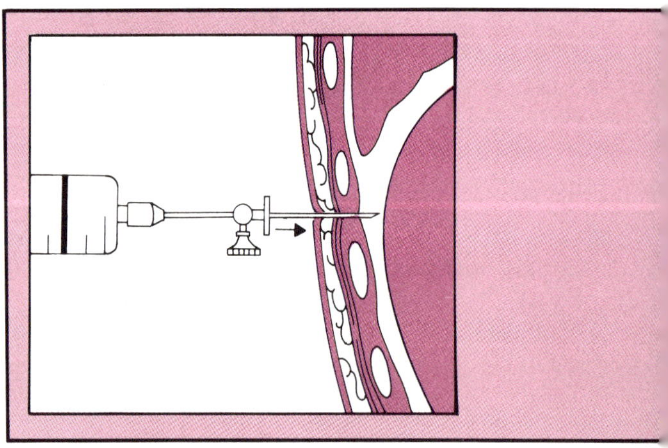

are picked up by cancerous tissue. A special machine then scans your body, providing doctors with images of individual organs or with cross sections of a particular part of the body. A scan identifies abnormal growths or changes in an organ's position caused by pressure from an abnormal growth.

Performed in the nuclear medicine department of a hospital, this test is usually referred to as a CAT or CT (computerized axial tomography) scan, but it may be called by other names as well. Another kind of scan, called a gallium scan, may be used for examining the thyroid, brain, bones, lungs, or entire body.

Ultrasound
Ultrasound is similar to radar. During an ultrasound test, high-frequency sound waves are bounced off a soft organ, like an eye or the heart. The echoes of the sound can be used to create a picture of the organ and will indicate any hard, abnormal lumps. This painless test isn't currently thought to have any lasting or dangerous side effects.

Limited surgery
In some surgical tests, a doctor will actually open up the patient and directly observe and even feel any organs he or she suspects are cancerous. More common, however, are the more limited surgical tests: biopsies and endoscopies.

Biopsy is a general term for any surgically obtained sample of tissue. A biopsy may be obtained in several ways:

- During surgery, for immediate analysis to see if the patient requires removal of all or part of an organ—often done during abdominal surgery.

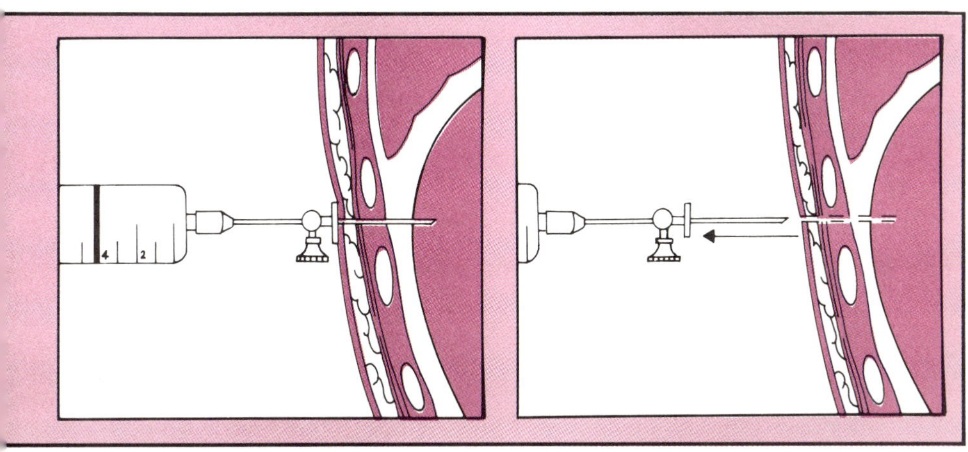

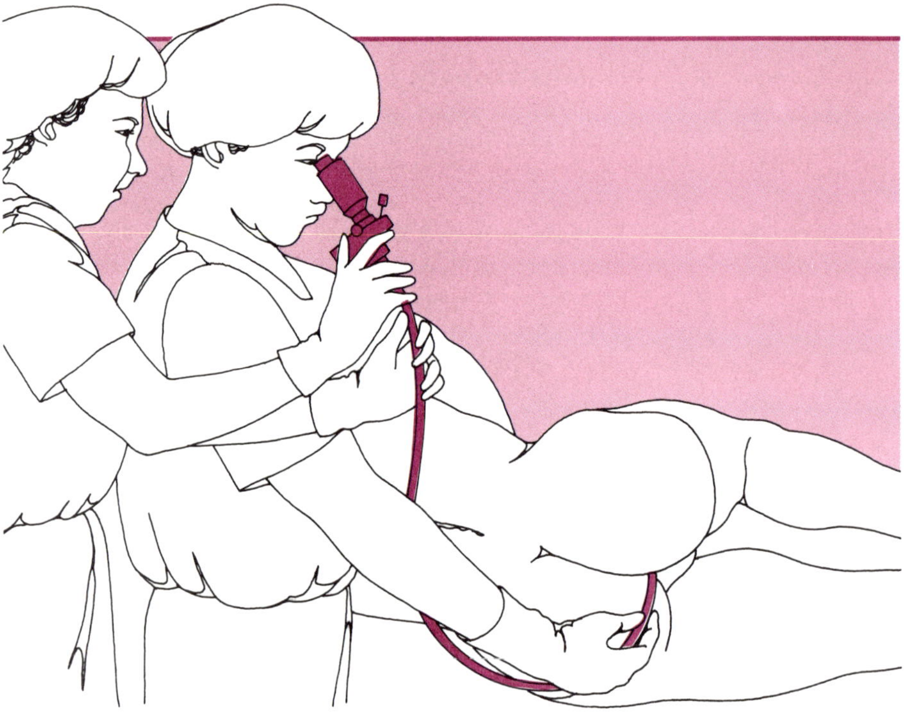

Endoscopy
In an endoscopy, the doctor passes a tube inside you and looks through it. He or she may also take a tissue sample at the same time.

- Through insertion of a hollow needle through the skin and into the organ in order to withdraw fluid containing cells to be studied; this is called an aspiration biopsy and is often done under local anesthesia to the lungs, liver, kidneys, breast, chest, or abdomen.
- Through an endoscope, a tube with a light attached and a special lens for viewing, through which the doctor can look into certain organs and take a biopsy.

Endoscopy is often used when your doctors suspect cancer of the lung, bladder, larynx, or digestive tract. It can be very uncomfortable. For example, to study the upper digestive tract, a doctor passes a tube down the esophagus; you would need a local anesthetic to prevent gagging. Different names identify different kinds of endoscopic procedures: sigmoidoscopy, which is endoscopy of the colon; laparoscopy, endoscopy of the abdomen; and bronchoscopy, endoscopy of the lungs, to name only three.

The biopsy is the final stage of cancer testing and yields the definitive diagnosis. A pathologist studies the tissue sample under a microscope, comparing it with normal tissue taken from the tumor margin. In general, the pathologist will study the tumor for changes in its tissue structure or in the appearance or arrangement of its cells; he or she will also check for migration of cells from one layer of tissue to another.

You'll probably never meet your pathologist, who's probably the most important person in diagnosing your cancer.

Besides these basic tests, others may be done on blood, urine, feces, and cells taken from smears and biopsies. These require little if any participation from you after the sample has been obtained, but they can teach doctors more about your case.

Staging the cancer

Once your doctors agree that you have cancer, they'll go to the next step in the diagnostic process: staging. Doctors must know the stage of a cancer so they can plan the best treatment. Staging is done after a biopsy: the doctor examines other tissues, organs, and lymph nodes to determine how much the cancer has spread, if at all. Each cancer is assigned to one of four stages:

- Stage I: The tumor is still localized to the site of origin.
- Stage II: The tumor has spread to nearby lymph nodes.
- Stage III: The tumor has spread to other organs, such as the lung, brain, liver, and bone. At this point cancer is thought of and treated as a disease that has spread throughout the body.
- Stage IV: Similar to Stage III, but refers to tumors with more complex patterns of spreading.

Staging may save the patient from unnecessary treatment. If the cancer is widespread, the patient needn't undergo extensive surgery or radiation, both of which are used primarily on people with localized cancer.

If you're told you have cancer: The psychological reaction

A serious illness is always a burden, but cancer carries with it a stigma that makes it different from any other disease. The tests, the treatments, the uncertain cure rates, the sudden possibility of imminent death or physical disfigurement—all take a profound toll on the patient's psyche. Then the patient most needs family, friends, and any other means of support.

Most patients' reactions to a cancer diagnosis have several common components. Each person's reaction will be influenced to some extent by age, sex, basic personality type, relationships with family and friends,

How cancer cells spread

Spreading through lymph system

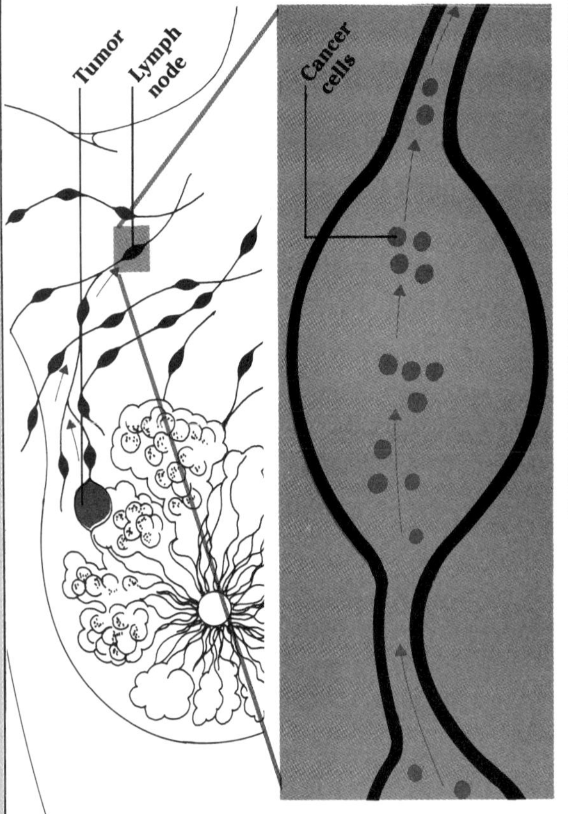

Spreading by direct invasion

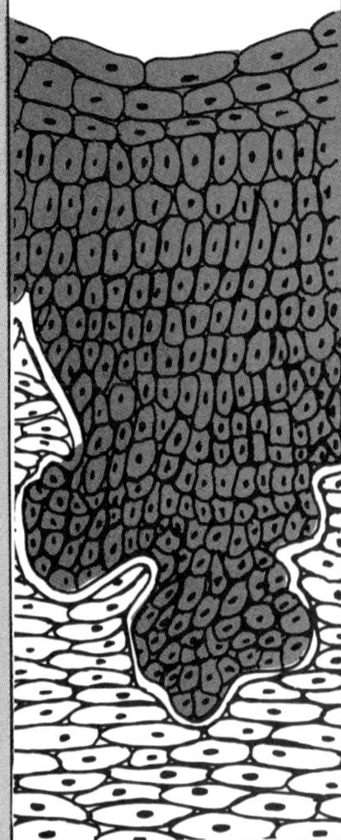

Cancer cells may take several routes when they spread to other parts of the body. Cells may break off from the original tumor and travel to other organs throughout the blood or lymph, or they may spread locally, within the same organ. Very rarely, cancer cells may spill from scalpels or other instruments used during tumor surgery. Certain tumors have characteristic spreading patterns: some lymph system tumors, for example, often spread to the lungs. If doctors suspect this, they may take a biopsy from any anticipated sites of spread, as well as from the original tumor site.

and individual beliefs. Even so, most patients experience at least the following emotions:

• Shock. When someone learns he or she has cancer, the initial shock is such that the person may actually forget where he or she is for a few seconds. The person may feel "unreal" or disoriented. If the patient isn't able to think clearly, details of the case shouldn't be discussed for a few days or even a week or two. Treatment can usually be delayed for that length of time with no ill effects.

The manifestations of shock
Different people express shock in different ways. Some people are visibly shaken, while others appear to react more calmly. A calm front, however, often hides very real fear and turmoil; it may also be a sign of denial. Friends and family may also be shocked to learn a loved one has cancer, and various expressions of shock on their part are to be expected.

• Denial. During denial, which follows closely after shock, the patient appears not to realize the seriousness of the disease. This is actually a normal, healthy, and important sign: it permits the patient to gather the emotional strength to confront the facts of the illness. It may also permit the person to remain levelheaded enough to cooperate with the doctors. Denial may become a serious problem, however, if the patient ignores the need for any necessary therapy.

• Guilt. This is a common reaction to a cancer diagnosis. A person may feel guilty because of personal habits, like smoking or poor eating habits, that may be related to the cancer. He or she may also feel guilty about being a burden on the family. Some patients feel that they've developed cancer as a punishment for some past sin.

• Depression. Depression may be caused by many things: fear of surgery, treatment, or death; and loss of physical integrity or self-esteem. No longer in control of the present or future, the patient must depend on doctors, nurses, and hospital staff for everything, sometimes even the most basic functions, like going to the bathroom. Privacy is rare: hospital patients seldom have a room to themselves; during tests people other than doctors and nurses may be present, which adds to the loss of privacy and self-respect. Many hospital procedures, including insertion of catheters (drains), administration of enemas, and gynecological and proctological examinations, would be an assault on anyone's dignity. Feelings of anger, fear, humiliation, and loss of self-worth may all manifest themselves as depression. This is a normal reaction, but some patients become pathologically depressed and may even lose the will to live. A prolonged refusal of food or medicine may be a severely depressed patient's attempt at suicide.

• Anger. An angry patient may direct his feelings at himself, family, friends, or hospital staff. This could be a healthy sign, if the patient can learn to direct anger at the disease and be more aggressive about seeking the best and safest treatment.

Is cancer contagious? *Cancer patients may feel isolated for another reason: friends and even family members may avoid them because they believe cancer is contagious. This fear is completely unfounded: even sexual intercourse with a cancer patient won't cause cancer in the partner. The strength with which this idea persists only reflects the grip that cancer has on the less rational parts of our minds.*

• Isolation. A patient may be reluctant to discuss either the disease or personal feelings, which in turn makes the person feel isolated from others. Family and friends often share this reluctance, either because they can't face the situation themselves or because they believe the patient would rather not talk about personal concerns.

The best way for you or anyone else to cope with any of these feelings is to talk about them. You'll find on page 93 a list of places to go for help and support. If you or a loved one has cancer, you're strongly urged to make use of that list. Sometimes a visit from the hospital chaplain can be comforting, or perhaps your priest, rabbi, or minister could be of help. Many communities have psychologists and social workers who specialize in the emotional care of seriously ill people; you might inquire about them. The hospital may have such an individual on call. These specialists can also promote communication among family members and friends. In addition, you may benefit from a talk with someone who's had the kind of cancer you have and has recovered and is leading a normal life.

Whatever the diagnosis, no cancer patient need suffer alone. As you know, cancer is a common disease. Its victims need as much help, understanding, and support as they can get, and they need to know that others around them have gone through the same kind of trauma and survived. The right frame of mind can improve the quality of each patient's remaining years and, some experts believe, may even influence the outcome of the treatment.

5 Treatment

Finding a second opinion
A good second opinion will confirm your diagnosis or offer you a different approach to treatment. Many insurance companies will pay for a second opinion; some even require it. But reputable doctors don't perform miracles, nor will they let you think they can. Don't get caught up in a search for the one doctor who'll tell you that you don't have cancer or that he or she can cure you completely, with no side effects.

One reason people fear cancer so much is that they fear the treatment for it. Cancer treatment can, in fact, be a grim experience and may involve loss of hair, limbs, or organs, as well as prolonged and debilitating side effects. But cancer treatment has come a long way over the past few decades, and doctors have become more and more sensitive to the terrible psychological toll it can take.

Surgery, radiation, and chemotherapy—the three standard ways of treating cancer—are continually being improved to minimize the possibility of devastating side effects. The search for drugs that can cure with the fewest possible complications is one of the hottest areas of cancer research today. According to experts at the National Institutes of Health, the ultimate goal of cancer treatment is a patient who's not only alive but *intact*: the cancer is either cured or in remission, and the patient looks and feels normal and can resume a normal life when treatment is over.

Still, treatment for cancer isn't pleasant. You can minimize the trauma somewhat by learning as much as you can about the treatment that's recommended for you, and what options may be available. Ask all the questions you want, and beware of any doctor who won't take the time to talk to you or who frowns on your getting another opinion. If a certain doctor makes you feel frightened or uncomfortable, find someone else. Good communication between cancer patients and those treating them is essential, so don't settle for a doctor just because a friend likes him or because she teaches at the local university. Find a doctor who'll answer your questions patiently and thoroughly: someone who you know will care about *you*.

Surgery

Surgery is the oldest method of treating cancer, and it's still the first choice of treatment for the most common cancers seen in this country. Not every operation is major surgery: some kinds of skin cancer, for example, can be removed in the doctor's office with a local anesthetic and a technique that amounts to little more than shaving the cancer off. Other kinds of cancer surgery, however, are major.

The legacy of cancer treatment

Among the most dreaded side effects of cancer treatment are mutilation and disfigurement. Radiation and chemotherapy often cause hair loss and skin problems, while surgery often means amputation or a basic change in essential bodily functions, as with an ostomy. An ostomy is an artificial opening in the abdominal wall through which urine or feces pass into a special drainage bag. Ostomies are done on patients who have surgery on the colon, rectum, or bladder. Colostomy and ileostomy are the most common ostomies performed.

Ostomy patients may at first feel horror and disgust at their condition. They can no longer eliminate normally: they must "go" into a bag that's always attached to them, and they must be careful to replace it at regular intervals. They might worry whether the ostomy bag will be detectable under their clothes and whether it will hinder their daily activities. In addition, they must care for the opening and keep it clean.

Yet living with an ostomy is handled perfectly well by thousands of patients who go to work, eat out, exercise regularly—in short, lead normal lives with one basic change in their routines. At first, each patient may have thought the condition unworkable, but, free of cancer, each made the adjustment.

The three kinds of cancer surgery are curative, preventive, and palliative. Doctors perform curative surgery to remove a tumor. Some growths aren't cancerous, but left in place, they will probably become so. For these, doctors use preventive surgery. Examples are removing a colon polyp or a skin lesion that may turn malignant. Palliative surgery relieves symptoms but doesn't cure the disease. Doctors perform palliative surgery to help incurable cancer patients suffer less. For example, an inoperable tumor may grow so large that it presses on a nerve and causes unbearable pain. By surgically cutting that nerve, doctors can relieve the patient's pain and greatly improve the quality of the patient's remaining life.

Curative surgery is best for treating localized, relatively small tumors like some found in the breast, lung, or colon. Doctors are now doing less surgery and relying more on chemotherapy and other forms of treatment that often yield better overall results. Tumors in the muscles or bones of the arms and legs used to be removed by amputating the entire limb; now, in many cases, a surgeon will simply cut out the tumor and treat the limb with radiation to kill any cancer cells that may remain.

Think things over
If you've been advised to have surgery, get two or three opinions before making a decision. Cancer surgery is rarely an emergency. You can take a week or two to think things over before you decide what kind of treatment you want and who should care for you.

Curative surgery is performed when doctors know they can remove the entire tumor during the operation. Tests are done to help determine as precisely as possible the tumor's size and extent before surgery, to make sure the operation won't be inadequate or unnecessary. Surgical techniques vary, depending on the tumor's size and location, but usually the surgeon removes all the visible tumor tissue along with a certain amount of the surrounding normal tissue and some nearby lymph nodes; they may contain cancer cells that have spread. This is often done all in one piece to avoid shedding any tumor cells into the open wound and is known as an "en bloc" resection or dissection. Because a few tumor cells might remain in the adjacent healthy tissue, en bloc surgery improves the chances of the patient's complete freedom from the cancer.

Other surgical techniques include:

• local excision: removal of the tumor only, which is adequate for most forms of skin cancer because they rarely spread to the lymph nodes

• electrosurgery: use of a high-frequency electrical current transmitted through a blade, needle, or disc electrode to cut or coagulate tissue; this is done for some skin, mouth, and rectum cancers

• cryosurgery: freezing and destroying a tumor with liquid nitrogen applied with a special probe; best for cancers of the brain, mouth, and prostate

• chemosurgery or Mohs' surgery: freezing and gradually shaving off the tumor until no more cancer tissue can be seen under a microscope; used with some skin cancers.

Many doctors now believe a biopsy shouldn't be part of major surgery. Combining the two was frequently done in the past, particularly for women with breast cancer—the woman would go into surgery for a biopsy and come out minus a breast. This unnecessary practice contributed to the trauma not only of surgery for breast cancer but of other kinds of cancer surgery as well.

The one exception to this recommendation is if you require abdominal surgery, as for colon cancer. This kind of surgery is particularly serious and complicated, so if doctors open up a patient for a biopsy that reveals the presence of cancer, they may remove the tumor at the same time to avoid making the patient undergo more major surgery almost at once.

Before surgery, your doctor will evaluate your general health, checking for things like:

- your ability to withstand the operation
- the likelihood of subsequent complications
- your nutritional state
- the health of your lungs
- the health of your heart.

If necessary, your doctor will take several days or even a week or more to improve your condition and get you into the best possible shape for surgery.

Side effects of surgery

As with all kinds of surgery, the greatest immediate danger of cancer surgery comes from the use of anesthesia. The three basic kinds of anesthesia are general,

Breast cancer surgery

Lumpectomy

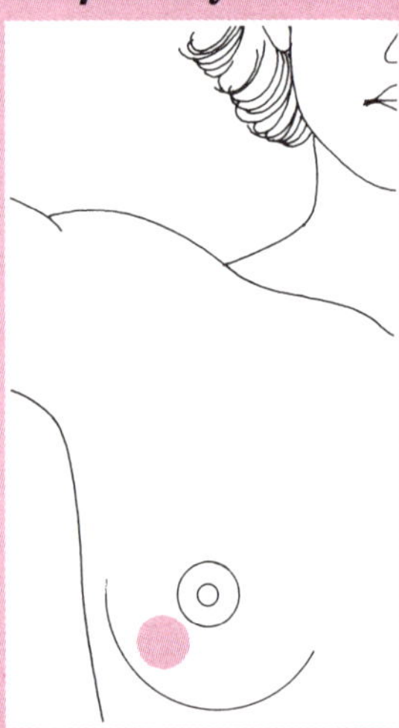

In the lumpectomy, also called a tumorectomy, only the tumor is removed. This procedure is a variation on a biopsy. Quadrantectomy and lumpectomy may be accompanied by chemotherapy, radiation, or both to kill any remaining tumor cells.

Quadrantectomy

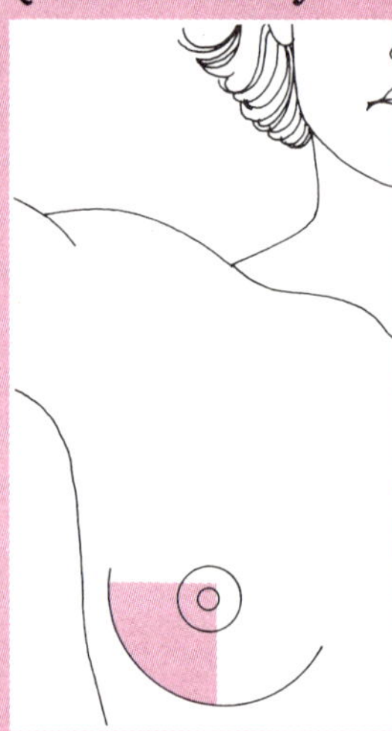

In the quadrantectomy, also called a partial or segmental mastectomy, the tumor is removed, along with some surrounding normal tissue and some skin and underlying muscle.

Simple mastectomy

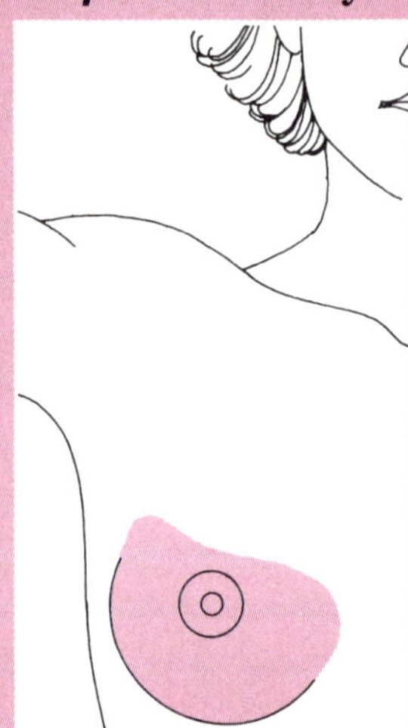

A simple mastectomy, also called a total or complete mastectomy, involves only removal of the breast, sometimes with a few lymph nodes.

local, and spinal. General anesthesia, the kind that lets you sleep during surgery, is used most often and carries a small but significant risk of affecting your breathing. Throughout the operation the anesthesiologist will sit at your head and monitor your vital signs, checking that the anesthetic is neither too light nor too deep. A local anesthetic is injected only into the area to be operated on, so you're awake during the operation. A local is used mostly for biopsies and for small, superficial tumors like skin tumors: it carries only a minimal risk of complications. A spinal anesthetic is injected near the spinal cord and results in numbness of the lower body from the area of injection to the toes. It is used on a variety of high-risk patients, particularly those who can't take inhaled anesthetics.

After surgery, doctors may place tubes in your nose or throat for a few hours or even days; these are mostly

Modified radical

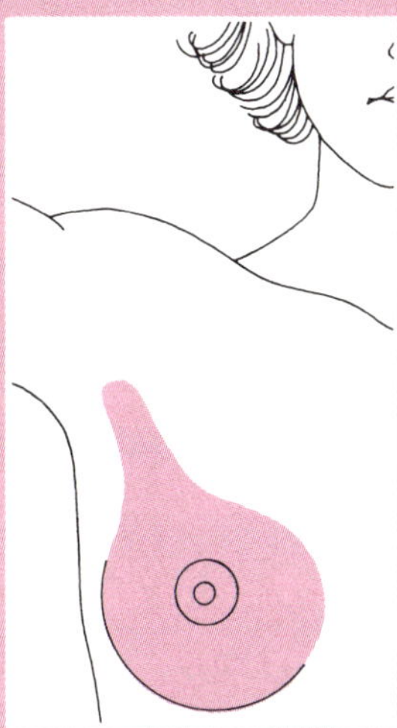

The modified radical mastectomy calls for removal of the breast, some of the lymph nodes, and, in some cases, removal of one of the chest muscles. While it still involves loss of a breast, recovery is easier than from a Halsted radical.

Halsted radical

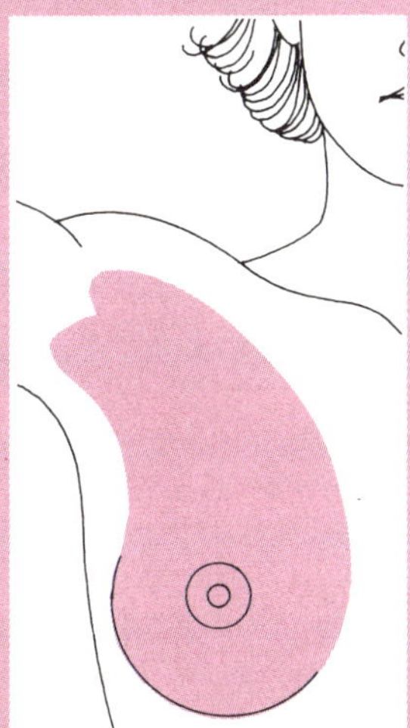

Halsted radical mastectomy involves removal of the breast, the underlying fat and chest muscles, the lymph nodes in the armpit, and sometimes even the bone in the arm. This operation was widely used until the late 1970s.

Artificial breast

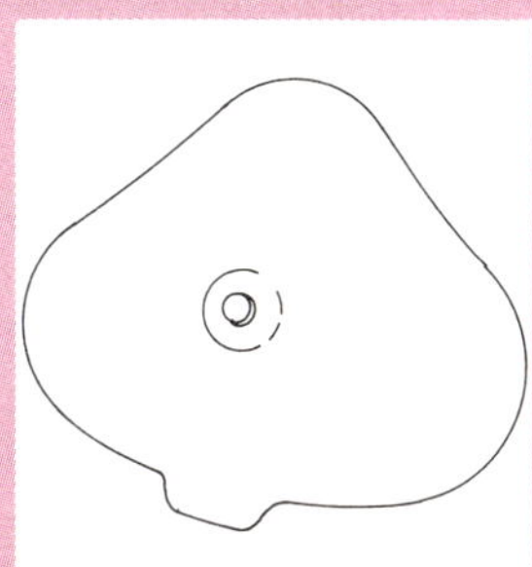

A woman who has had a radical or simple mastectomy can be fitted for an artificial breast that looks entirely natural. The one pictured here is called the Second to Nature breast. A woman can insert it in the cup of a bra or attach it with adhesive to the chest skin. Many patients like its convenience, ease of care, and realistic appearance. Check with your doctor before trying it, however.

What to do and what to avoid after a mastectomy

With the removal of lymph nodes and lymph vessels in a radical mastectomy, your arm may swell, and the body's ability to fight infection in that arm will be greatly reduced. The following list of what to do and what to avoid will help you prevent complications.	***Do***	***Avoid***
	• Contact your doctor if the affected arm becomes red, warm, or unusually hard or swollen. • Protect the hand and arm on the affected side. • Order and wear a Medic Alert tag engraved: Caution —lymphedema arm—no tests—no injections. • Use a thimble while sewing. • Wear a loose rubber glove while washing dishes. • Stay out of strong sunlight. • Apply lanolin hand cream several times a day.	*• Injury to cuticles or hangnails • Strong detergents • Reaching into a hot oven • Cuts, bruises, insect bites • Digging in the garden or working near thorny bushes • Having blood drawn; injections • Having a blood pressure cuff applied • Wearing jewelry or a wristwatch • Carrying heavy bags or purse.*

to help you breathe. If you've had surgery on your digestive tract, you won't be able to eat and will be fed through an intravenous (I.V.) tube for a while. Expect to feel some pain from your wound: this is normal and subsides within a week.

Options in breast cancer surgery

The age of doing radical surgery for breast cancer has passed. Now the modified radical mastectomy has become the most widely used procedure, and more emphasis is given to reconstructive surgery.

Implants offer mastectomy patients even more options. Safe, natural-looking silicone implants are now available, and many doctors get good results with implants made from a woman's own skin and muscle taken from other parts of her body. Sometimes a new breast can be created, and sometimes all that's needed is a new nipple, which can also be provided. This kind of surgery can often be done simultaneously with the mastectomy, allowing the woman to avoid the trauma of seeing herself without a breast.

Emotional trauma

Another kind of side effect from cancer surgery is widespread and difficult to treat: emotional trauma. It comes from disfigurement from head or neck surgery, removal of a breast, limb, or larynx, or the change in body function that follows removal of the colon or bladder. Patients may have to adjust to profound changes in physical appearance and in the most basic aspects of their lives: how they walk, talk, eat, and pass wastes. Only sustained emotional support from friends, family, and hospital staff can help these patients come to grips with their new condition.

Dissection and resection: What's the difference?
Dissection *is a general term that refers to the orderly cutting of tissue to separate and observe anatomical parts. It doesn't necessarily mean anything will be removed.* Resection *is more specific and means that tissue will be removed during the procedure. In many states, laws now require doctors to tell cancer patients about all the treatment methods available to them and to fully explain the results, advantages, and disadvantages of each one.*

Here are two recommended procedures:

- Arrange for the patient to talk to others who've been through similar operations.
- Contact one of the nationwide support networks that send volunteers into hospitals or that meet the patient outside the hospital after discharge.

Cancer treatment is improving all the time, and that's of first importance. Nearly as vital, though, is emotional support for patients.

Radiation therapy

Perhaps half of all cancer patients receive radiation therapy at some point in their treatment. This therapy involves the use of high-energy radiation to disrupt a cancer cell's DNA, thus interfering with cell division. The reasoning behind radiation therapy is that cancer cells are more vulnerable to the effects of radiation than normal cells because cancer cells divide more quickly.

Like surgery, radiation therapy can be either curative or palliative. And, as with surgery, it works best on tumors that are still fairly localized. Curative radiation is used most often in cases where surgery might be too disfiguring, as with cancers of the head and neck. For example, radiation cures 90 percent of the early cases of laryngeal cancer without removal of the larynx, which means the patient's normal voice is saved. Surgery can also cure this form of cancer, but at the expense of the patient's voice. Cervical cancers and some kinds of skin cancer also respond well to radiation therapy. It's also used for treating Hodgkin's disease (cancer of the lymph glands), and for tumors that may be too big to be surgically removed.

Radiation is administered in units called rads. A total dose of 3,000 rads is considered low; 6,000 to 8,000 rads is a high dose. Doses can be given either internally or externally. Internal radiation is a way of delivering a highly concentrated amount of radiation to the tumor while minimizing exposure to the surrounding tissue. It calls for implanting a source of radiation, usually radium or cesium, at the tumor site—for example, the cervix or uterus. The implant remains in the hospitalized patient 2 or 3 days; guests are limited to the immediate family (pregnant women are excluded), who should stay no longer than 30 minutes a day and sit at least 5 feet away. Doctors and nurses also must limit their visits to 30 minutes. After that, the radiation source is removed and visits are no longer restricted.

External radiation therapy is used more often. This involves exposure to brief periods of radiation, similar to getting an X-ray. Each treatment may last 2 to 5 minutes and is done 4 or 5 times a week for 2 to 4 weeks. The treatments are painless, and uninvolved organs are protected by lead shields placed on the patient's body.

How radiation works on cancer cells

Radiation affects the way cells grow and reproduce. By damaging growth elements in cells, it has a vital effect on cancer cells because cancer cells reproduce so much faster than normal cells.

Because X-rays can damage all cells, the technician will irradiate the area of the cancer only.

Side effects of radiation therapy

The purpose of radiation therapy is to attack and kill rapidly dividing tumor cells. In theory, tumor cells are more susceptible than normal cells to these attacks, but, in fact, normal tissue also sustains some radiation damage.

Radiation equipment has improved greatly over the past 15 to 20 years: previously, doctors had to use equipment that delivered low-voltage radiation that couldn't be accurately aimed at the tumor and didn't penetrate the skin well. This often resulted in the serious skin burns that many people still associate with radiation treatment. Today's equipment produces high-energy beams that penetrate the skin efficiently and can be aimed at tumors with great accuracy, thus decreasing the possibility of serious burns. Today's patients also receive radiation much earlier in their treatment, when they're still healthy enough to tolerate its effects; formerly, it was used as a last resort on patients who were already seriously ill. As doctors have become more skillful at using radiation, they've learned to determine how much radiation normal tissues can withstand without excessive complications, and they've learned which tumors will and won't respond to radiation in reasonable doses. If radiation can't destroy a tumor in a dose that doesn't do excessive damage to normal cells, it won't be used.

Nevertheless, radiation may still cause serious side effects. These occur mostly in organs that have rapidly dividing cell populations: the skin, hair, digestive tract, bladder, and bone marrow. Prior to receiving any radiation treatment, you'll be evaluated carefully for your capacity to withstand the radiation's effects. Remember that different people vary greatly in their response to radiation and that side effects depend upon the dose received and the site and size of the area radiated. Almost everyone experiences some side effects from radiation, but many patients can lead normal lives while undergoing treatment. Others, unfortunately, may become more seriously ill. Still, when all details and options are outlined by a doctor, many patients decide that the side effects are tolerable if the cancer can ultimately be eliminated.

Some general radiation sickness occurs in nearly everyone, to varying degrees. Symptoms include fatigue, nausea, vomiting, headache, and loss of appetite. Drugs can be given to relieve the nausea and vomiting, if necessary. Other side effects occur in the part of the body that gets the radiation and may include:

- head and neck: temporary hair loss; dryness, soreness, or inflammation of the mouth and throat; pain on eating or swallowing; loss of taste
- chest: soreness of the esophagus, pain on swallowing, a dry cough, shortness of breath
- upper abdomen: nausea, vomiting, appetite loss
- lower abdomen: bowel irritation that may cause cramps and/or watery diarrhea; bladder irritation that may cause painful or frequent urination and bloody urine; in women, radiation to the ovaries may cause sterility and premature menopause; in men, radiation to the testicles may cause sterility
- skin: redness (like a sunburn), tanning, blistering, poor wound healing in radiated area
- bone marrow: this is where red and white blood cells are made, so radiation may lower the blood count of these cells; the patient may become anemic or prone to bleeding disorders; decreased white blood cells make the patient more susceptible to infection.

Later effects of radiation may not occur until months or even years after the treatment. These result from damage to blood vessels, which can no longer properly nourish the tissues they inhabit, and include:

- difficulty swallowing due to esophageal scarring
- dry mouth and tooth damage due to scarring of the salivary glands

Try a soft diet

While undergoing radiation therapy, you may experience digestive problems. If so, try some of the foods listed on this sample menu; they're less taxing on your digestive system.

Breakfast

1/2 cup orange juice
1/2 cup farina
1 soft-cooked egg
1 slice enriched white toast
2 teaspoons butter or margarine
1/2 cup whole milk
1 cup coffee

Lunch

3 ounces ground chicken
1 small baked potato (no skin)
1/2 cup pureed asparagus
1/2 cup canned cherries
1 soft roll
2 teaspoons butter or margarine
1 cup whole milk
1 cup tea
2 teaspoons sugar

Dinner

1/2 cup cream of mushroom soup
3 ounces ground beef
1 mashed potato
1/2 cup pureed or diced carrots
1 scoop vanilla ice cream
1 slice light rye bread
2 teaspoons butter or margarine
1/2 cup whole milk
1 cup coffee
2 teaspoons sugar

• high blood pressure or kidney failure due to kidney scarring. Radiation may also raise the patient's risk of developing leukemia or a new tumor in the radiated area.

The best person to administer radiation therapy is a board-certified radiation oncologist. This is a doctor who's had at least 3 years' experience in treating cancer with radiation and has passed a written examination that documents his or her expertise. The radiation oncologist often works with a patient's doctor to deliver the best possible care to the patient. Don't confuse this specialist with a board-certified radiologist, who specializes in performing diagnostic X-rays. Some radiologists may be experts in treating cancer, but ensure yourself the best care by finding a board-certified radiation oncologist.

Foods to avoid

If you're experiencing trouble digesting food as a result of radiation therapy, you may want to avoid the following foods: tough, fibrous meat, whole sliced meat or poultry, whole frankfurters, shrimp or lobster, scallops, all cheeses except ricotta, cream cheese, and cottage cheese, fried eggs, coarse breads or rolls with seeds, hard rolls, raisins, nuts, raw vegetables, and the spices and raw fruits you cannot tolerate.

Chemotherapy

Chemotherapy involves the administration of drugs or hormones in the form of pills, injections, or intravenous infusion. Since they enter the bloodstream, these chemicals reach all the body's tissues and are best for treating widespread cancers like leukemia and Hodgkin's disease. Chemotherapy has enabled doctors to cure cancers that were considered incurable only a few years ago. It can also be used for palliation and as adjuvant (auxiliary) therapy, meaning it's administered after all the visible tumor has been removed, in the hope of destroying any small cell clusters that might remain.

The basic principle behind chemotherapy is similar to that guiding radiation therapy: the drugs damage both normal and cancer cells, but normal cells are better able to repair themselves, while cancer cells are killed. Chemotherapy is often administered as a "cocktail" of several different drugs: if each drug has a different side effect, all can be administered in fairly large doses for maximal cancer destruction. This kind of aggressive therapy is performed only when doctors believe that they can achieve a cure, because its side effects can be serious. If your doctors suggest combination chemotherapy, ask questions about its value for your case. Thinking your cancer is curable, they will treat it with the highest drug doses you can tolerate, even if this increases the likelihood of side effects. Such treatment may continue for up to a year if the cancer reacts as your doctors planned. Many patients decide the price is worth paying if they're cured.

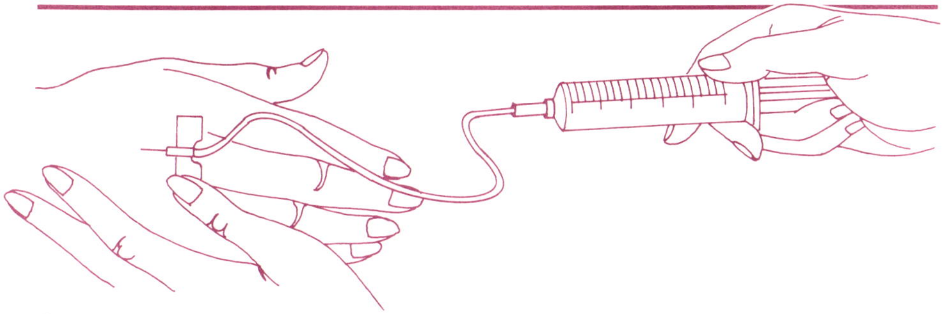

Chemotherapy
One method of giving chemotherapy is through a needle or catheter placed in the hand. After the drug has been administered, the needle will be removed.

Palliative chemotherapy is usually administered in smaller doses, since doctors aren't trying to destroy the cancer. It's had good results in relieving the symptoms of tumors of the breast, prostate, thyroid, kidney, ovary, uterus, and lung, among others.

Adjuvant chemotherapy is highly controversial. Some doctors feel it's not always necessary, since they're not always certain that any cancer cells are left after surgery or radiation. They question whether patients should be subjected to the side effects of chemotherapy unless absolutely necessary. Currently, adjuvant chemotherapy seems to work best on children's cancers, and it's being tested on breast cancer patients, where it may prolong lives.

If chemotherapy has been recommended for you, you may want to ask your doctor these questions:

- Will it cure me, prolong my life, or make me feel better?

- What are the side effects and how severe will they be?

- If I receive palliative chemotherapy, when is the best time for me to get it: when I still feel all right, in the hopes that it will prolong my life even if it causes side effects, or when my disease starts causing me pain and other kinds of discomfort?

Side effects of chemotherapy

As with radiation side effects, chemotherapy side effects occur mostly in parts of the body that have the most rapidly growing cell populations: the skin, hair, digestive tract, and bone marrow, among others. Here, too, side effects vary widely from person to person. Some people experience only very mild discomfort and are able to lead normal lives while undergoing chemotherapy; others have side effects that are severe enough to hospitalize them. Much depends on your overall health, the kind of cancer you have, which drugs you receive, and whether you receive them individually or in combination.

The most common side effects are those of the digestive tract: nausea, vomiting, loss of appetite, diarrhea, mouth sores, and blood in the stool. Drugs can usually control the nausea and vomiting. Other side effects may occur in the following organs:

- Skin: damage to skin or soft tissue may occur if a drug given intravenously leaks out of the vein. This can lead to painful sores or skin ulcers. Tell the doctor or nurse who gives you the injection if the injection hurts or burns. Chemotherapy may also cause a rash, redness, skin discoloration, itching, or peeling. These effects can be relieved with drugs and usually subside after chemotherapy.
- Bone marrow: suppression of bone marrow cell division may cause anemia and subsequent weakness and fatigue; abnormal bleeding that may require transfusions; and increased susceptibility to infections. A patient's blood count should be monitored during chemotherapy.
- Sexual organs: temporary or permanent sterility in both men and women; vaginal dryness or soreness; cessation of menstrual periods; cessation of sperm production; uncertain risk to future children due to possible DNA damage. In pregnant women, fetal damage may occur, especially during the first 3 months of pregnancy; some doctors even recommend therapeutic abortion if chemotherapy must be done at this time.
- Neuromuscular: weakness, possible paralysis; fatigue; occasional tingling in hands and feet; rare clumsiness and loss of balance; soreness and itching of eyes; constipation; numbness in fingers.
- Hair: hair loss is often temporary, but hair may grow in thinner and finer than before; associated with only some of the drugs used in chemotherapy.

Chemotherapy drugs may interact with other drugs to give unexpected side effects. Ask your doctor before you take any other drugs while you're on chemotherapy.

Some of the drugs used in chemotherapy may be carcinogenic, which means they may cause a new cancer at some future date. Many doctors and their patients feel that this risk is worth taking. However, younger patients are frequently warned against having adjuvant chemotherapy because the long-term effects of chemotherapy drugs are still unknown.

Treatments to prevent hair loss

Your doctor may try to control your hair loss in one of two ways. He or she may use a tourniquet (as shown) or he or she may use ice applied to your scalp. Both methods slow the blood flow into your head during the chemotherapy treatment.

Good news about children with leukemia

The survival rate of children with leukemia has increased dramatically as a result of improvements in chemotherapy treatment. In just ten years, the survival rate for white children with acute lymphocytic leukemia has increased from 4 percent to 65 percent. In some medical centers, the percentage of children surviving with acute lymphocytic leukemia is up to 75 percent. Continuing research in 80 U.S. medical centers yields new and better drugs for treatment.

If the chemotherapy you require is relatively simple and nontoxic, your family doctor or nurse may administer it. More dangerous or complicated drugs should be administered by a board-certified medical oncologist, a specialist with several years' training in internal medicine and adult cancer medicine. If a child needs chemotherapy, treatment should be by a pediatric oncologist. Both these doctors specialize in cancer chemotherapy and are qualified to direct all aspects of a cancer patient's care.

Experimental treatments

Scientists around the world are seeking a cancer cure that will be fast, painless, and devoid of side effects. While several research avenues look promising, responsible researchers always warn that years of tests are necessary before a new cancer treatment can ethically be offered to patients. A substance that looks promising during early research may later prove disappointing. One such substance is interferon.

First discovered in 1957, interferon is produced by the body as part of its defense system against viral infection. When researchers found that interferon slows down the division of cancer cells, some of them hailed it as the long-awaited "miracle cure": a drug that destroys cancer but leaves normal tissue alone, thus having few, if any, side effects. After the excitement died down, however, scientists found that the interferon story wasn't all that simple. First of all, human cancer cells could be destroyed only by human interferon, which was difficult to obtain and prohibitively expensive. With the advent of new technology, scientists produced interferon by transplanting human interferon

How interferon destroys cancer
This drawing shows how interferon stimulates an immune response that kills malignant cells.

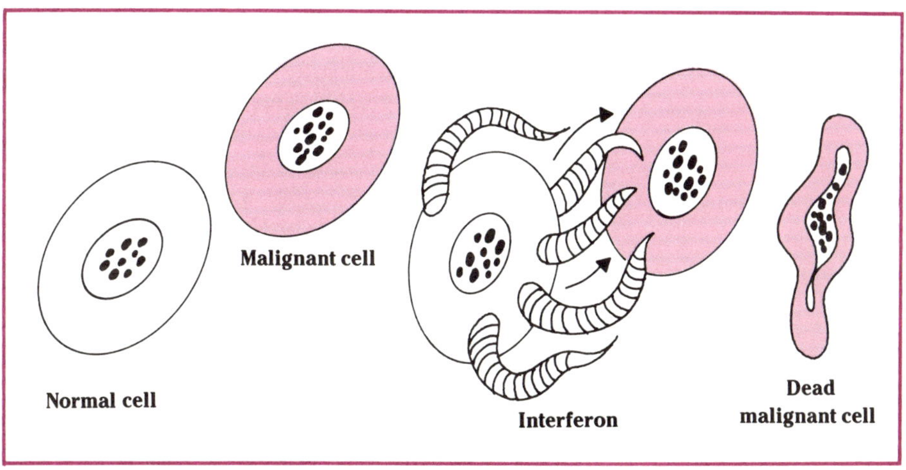

genes into bacteria, which then became little interferon factories. Unfortunately, this recombinant interferon, as it was called, turned out to be slightly different from true human interferon, and recombinant interferon may not be as effective as the natural kind. Because animal studies have yielded promising results, doctors continue to test interferon against human cancers of the lung, brain, kidney, breast, and larynx, as well as malignant melanoma. Interferon can be administered while patients receive radiation or chemotherapy. Its side effects, such as headache, fever, fatigue, rash, weight loss, and a lowered white blood cell count, seem less severe than those caused by chemotherapy drugs. In short, interferon still holds a lot of promise as a cancer treatment, but scientists won't know enough about it for years to include it in their standard arsenal of cancer weapons.

Another experimental treatment

Hyperthermia—the opposite of hypothermia—offers another experimental way to fight cancer. Higher than normal body temperatures are applied to tumors to kill them. This technique is related to the body's natural fever mechanism.

In 1975 researchers at the Memorial Sloan-Kettering Cancer Center in New York found a second, interferon-related chemical that has since created great excitement as a possible cancer treatment. Tumor necrosis factor, or TNF, is produced by human immune cells that have been exposed to bacteria. It prevents cancer cell growth and kills cancer cells by breaking their walls. Testing of the necrosis factor in humans has begun only recently, but in animals it seems to control cancer with few adverse effects. TNF has been tested on 62 kinds of human cancer tumors grown in laboratories, and it killed or inhibited cell growth in 40 of those tumors. So far it seems most effective against bone tumors and certain tumors of the breast and colon.

TNF belongs to the same chemical family as interferon, and when the two substances are combined, they're more effective than either one alone. As with interferon, TNF holds great promise as a cancer treatment, but years of testing remain.

Many other cancer treatments are currently being tested. One, called immunotherapy, involves stimulating the body's own defense system to fight tumor cells and to repair the damage done by both the disease and the methods used to treat it. A second technique, hyperthermia, raises the temperature around the tumor or in the patient's body to kill cancer cells. This, too, has shown some promise. As scientists learn more, they can use that knowledge to improve and devise cancer treatments lacking the devastating side effects that so many people fear.

6

Avoiding quack cures

Caution
Suspect a quack when you hear words like nonstandard, unorthodox, nontoxic, completely natural, unproven treatment.

Mr. Smith was frightened. A few days earlier he'd noticed a lump in his right testicle, which turned out to be a tumor that had already spread to several other organs. He'd been referred to a medical oncologist for chemotherapy and was now in that doctor's office, listening to him.

"I'm going to start you on a high-dose regimen of chemotherapy, using a combination of drugs," the doctor said. "Because the doses are so high, you'll probably have some pretty severe side effects: probably nausea, vomiting, and muscle pain. I can give you narcotics for the pain, but if the side effects become bad enough, you may need to be hospitalized. You may feel bad, but that won't necessarily mean the chemotherapy isn't working. Your chances of cure are about fifty percent. If the chemotherapy doesn't work, you have about a year." Mr. Smith was 30 years old.

Understandably depressed, Mr. Smith repeated this conversation to a friend, who said, "Don't be upset. Most of these medical guys are out for money. My brother-in-law had the same condition you do, and he found a clinic in Mexico that specialized in treating cancer patients with diet therapy. They cured Sam in a month, with no side effects, and he looks great now. It also cost about one-tenth of what these doctors charge. Forget the chemotherapy: go to Mexico." What would you do?

Mr. Smith isn't real, but he's typical of the thousands of cancer patients who, each year, seek out what some doctors diplomatically call "unproven" treatments, administered by people less diplomatically known as quacks. Quacks prey on the fear, suffering, and uncertainty of patients and their families. They take advantage of the fact that most people know very little about how their bodies work and even less about how cancer develops and spreads. These practitioners describe their treatments as "alternative," "nonstandard," "unorthodox," or "nontoxic." Conventional doctors call them unproven because they've been either inadequately tested or tested and found useless. Standard methods of treating cancer have been subjected to years of testing, and their efficacy against certain kinds of cancer is known. This doesn't mean they're all proven cures, but that doctors know what kinds of results to expect from them. Unfortunately, most cancer treatment is, at best, unpleasant, so if you hear about a new treatment that's free of side effects and 100 percent guaranteed to work, you may be strongly tempted. You should resist.

A theory of contamination
Metabolic therapy proponents use special diets, internal irrigation, and spiritual attitudes to cleanse and purify the body since they believe cancer comes from inadequate elimination of wastes.

Detoxification
Proponents of this remedy claim that cancer is caused by toxins, or poisons, in the body. If the body is cleansed, or "detoxified," the cancer will go away. Toward this end, detoxification experts may prescribe special diets, sweat baths, enemas, and other remedies, all designed to rid the body of cancer. This treatment doesn't work.

The appeal of the quack

Some reasons people may turn to quack remedies include:

• Desperate patients may feel they have nothing to lose by trying the unproven treatment, especially if they've been told they're going to die anyway.

• Some people mistrust doctors and organized medicine; they prefer "natural" remedies like herbs, fruits, and vegetables.

• Quacks often make their sales pitches in highly emotional terms; they'll refer to surgery, radiation, and chemotherapy as "cutting, burning, and poisoning," making frightening therapies sound even worse.

• Quacks capitalize on the shortcomings of conventional medicine, which emphasizes cure over care; many doctors project an impatient or unsympathetic attitude and are relatively ignorant about supportive therapies like nutrition.

• Some patients want to try every possible means of treatment, so they may try an unproven treatment while they're on standard therapy; an understanding doctor won't object to this, but if the patient doesn't improve, the quack will blame this failure on the conventional treatment.

• Quack cures *are* often cheaper than orthodox therapies: regular cancer care may cost anywhere from $20,000 to $100,000, while an unproven remedy may cost about $2,000. This isn't, however, covered by insurance.

Laetrile

Also known as nitriloside or Vitamin B_{17}, laetrile is made from a substance called amygdalin, which comes from apricot pits. Amygdalin has a cyanide component attached to it; this is what supposedly kills the cancer cells. Without question, cyanide is poisonous, and people have poisoned themselves with laetrile. What's more, no one has found any evidence to support the use of laetrile against cancer. Nonetheless, each year 50,000 to 75,000 Americans ask for treatment with it. Many regular doctors ask that, if you must try laetrile, at least try conventional therapy first. Why? Because the valuable treatment time that you waste may cost you dearly.

Vitamin C is controversial

Unlike laetrile or metabolic therapy, Vitamin C is controversial even though it has unquestioned benefits, like assisting the body during stress, helping heal wounds, and aiding the immune system. Even so, none of those good effects proves that Vitamin C can control cancer.

Nutritional or metabolic therapy

This kind of treatment relies on the use of diets and nutritional supplements to cure cancer. It may consist of having the patient drink prescribed amounts of vegetable juice and follow a special diet with or without large doses of vitamins, minerals, and other compounds. None of this may be harmful—cancer patients do have important nutritional needs—but nutritional therapy alone can't cure cancer.

Vitamin C has become highly controversial in cancer treatment, largely because its effects have been promoted by one of this century's most eminent scientists, Linus Pauling. Dr. Pauling and his supporters claim that Vitamin C can control or cure cancer in patients whose white blood cells haven't been affected by radiation or chemotherapy. They maintain that tests disproving Vitamin C's effects aren't valid because they were done on patients whose immune systems (the white blood cells) had already been impaired by conventional treatment methods. Scientists at the Mayo Clinic have risen to Dr. Pauling's challenge by testing Vitamin C on patients with colon cancer who hadn't been treated with radiation or chemotherapy. They've found that Vitamin C has no effect, although Dr. Pauling has responded that it wasn't administered long enough. The debate rages on, but for now most carefully conducted studies haven't demonstrated any curative effect of Vitamin C over cancer.

Devices

Contraptions that allegedly cure cancer come and go. One of the most recent was the orgone box: a zinc-lined box in which the patient sat to absorb orgone energy, which fights the tumor. In fact, the box served only one purpose: to earn money for its promoters. Certain charms, necklaces, and bracelets also appear occasionally on the scene as supposed cancer cures; most disappear quickly.

How to recognize a quack

Today's charlatans are vastly different from the hawkers of snake oil who used to peddle their wares in small towns and at country fairs. They may call themselves doctors, wear white coats, work in lavish clinics, and have offices whose walls contain rows of impressive-looking diplomas. Still, be suspicious of "doctors" who:

Have an unusual degree after their names, such as D.N. (doctor of naturopathy), or D.M. (doctor of metaphysics); these degrees usually come from mail-order diploma mills or unaccredited universities.

Claim their "research" was too imaginative or avant-garde to be conducted at a well-known laboratory, so it was done at an independent laboratory instead.

Rely on anecdotes or testimonials, often from people who may be famous but know nothing about medicine, instead of sharing their findings with other scientists by publishing in professional journals or attending scientific meetings.

Claim to have one secret remedy for all forms of cancer.

Promise sure success with no side effects.

Don't confirm a cancer diagnosis with a biopsy, which is the only sure way to know if someone really has cancer; thus, you may be "cured"—but you may never have had cancer to begin with.

Rely on unorthodox tests.

Have flamboyant, charismatic personalities and use emotional and pseudoscientific language ("cutting, burning, and poisoning").

May use both conventional and unconventional methods of treatment but, if unsuccessful, blame the conventional treatment.

Accuse the medical establishment of persecuting them and often compare themselves to famous scientists of the past who were persecuted due to ignorance and prejudice.

Claim the medical establishment is greedy and run by a conspiracy of doctors, drug companies, and the government.

Keep poor records, if any, so their data can't be checked by anyone else.

The danger of unproven treatment

You may wonder, if these treatments don't hurt patients who're looking for something more, what's the harm in trying them? The biggest tragedy occurs if patients have an early form of cancer that can be cured, but waste valuable time on worthless remedies. By the time they visit a regular doctor, their disease may be much more advanced. The worst side effect of unproven treatment, then, may be unnecessary suffering.

A natural poison
Laetrile produces cyanide, a poison that comes from such foods as apricots, plums, peaches, lima beans, almonds, and cloves. Laetrile supporters argue that the cyanide kills cancer cells by reacting to an enzyme they contain. Laetrile can cause high blood pressure, vomiting, and dizziness—and furthermore, it's toxic.

The relationship between you and your doctor may also be irrevocably damaged if you decide to seek an unconventional cure. If it doesn't work, you may feel too guilty and embarrassed to come back; your doctor may also feel guilty, as well as angry and frustrated. Ideally, your doctor should keep an open mind. If you insist on trying an unproven treatment, your doctor should encourage your continued communication, including your return for regular treatment. Best of all, perhaps, you and your doctor should continue with your conventional treatment while exploring other treatment options.

If you're tempted to try an unproven treatment on yourself or a loved one, discuss it with your doctor first. If your doctor proves narrow-minded or unsympathetic, change doctors before you change treatments. Learn all you can about the treatment you're considering, not just from material by the practitioner and his or her supporters, but from objective accounts, if you can find any.

And remember: doctors and their families get cancer, too. When they do, they use the same treatments they prescribe for their patients.

7

After treatment

Keep lines of communication open
One thing patients don't need is to be "protected" from the reality of their condition. Lies and evasion simply increase feelings of resentment and isolation. They also shut down the lines of communication that must remain open. Furthermore, if patients want to make realistic plans for the future, they must know how sick they are and what they can anticipate in the weeks, months, or years to come.

Cancer can take a devastating toll on all aspects of a patient's life: personal relationships, career, identity, appearance. The cured patient who returns home must resume a place in the family and a role in society, often in the face of significant financial and emotional pressures. The family that has learned to make do must now readjust to having the patient back, sometimes with profound changes in appearance or physical needs. Terminal patients have a different set of needs: should they live out their last days at home, in a hospital, or in a hospice? How can they best provide for those they're leaving behind? And, most important, how do they cope with the knowledge that they're going to die?

Special needs of cancer patients

All cancer patients share certain basic needs. Other needs differ from one patient to the next, depending on individual circumstances. Their loved ones have needs, too, as they learn to live with—or without—someone who is, or has been, seriously ill. Cancer doesn't go away when the tumor disappears: its repercussions are felt by all involved for years afterward, often for the rest of their lives.

For all cancer patients and those who love them, the most important needs are for support and communication. Maintaining good communication can make the difference between relationships preserved or destroyed, lives wasted or fulfilled, memories cherished or repressed. Almost everyone benefits from professional help at this time, and no one should feel embarrassed about seeking it.

Patients also need to know that, for as long as they live, they will remain integral parts of their families. People don't always have to speak their emotions; sometimes touching, hugging, or holding hands is all that's needed to reassure a sick person.

At the same time, patients must be encouraged to remain independent for as long as possible. No one benefits when family members start catering to one person. Having the illness is hard enough; many people don't like to be reminded that they can't do everything they used to do, even if their disability is only temporary. And family members themselves may grow to resent a patient they feel must be waited on. An independent patient will be able to resume normal life that much faster.

Remain active
Above all, patients should be encouraged to take control of their well-being by helping themselves as much as possible. This might mean attending group discussions, seeking help from hospital social workers and moral support from the family, returning to work as soon as possible, and remaining as active as they can in the outside interests they enjoyed before becoming cancer patients. Patients can also help themselves by maintaining normal relationships and by discussing their disease openly, instead of trying to protect others by hiding it.

Finally, all patients need a close relationship with their doctors. Good emotional support is as important a part of cancer treatment as good medical care. The devastating impact of the disease, its treatment, and its aftermath are softened considerably when patients and their families have access to doctors who understand their needs, encourage communication, and answer their questions honestly. In their reluctance to discuss their disease with others, many patients also come to depend entirely on their doctors for communication and support. In this case, the relationship is even more important. The doctor needn't be someone who's directly involved with the patient's cancer treatment, but he or she should know the patient and be familiar with the case. Sometimes a family practitioner or internist is the best choice. The doctor should be available around the clock and should be able to talk to the patient about fears of illness or death (many doctors aren't able to do this). He or she should also encourage the patient to learn all about the illness and to ask any questions that come to mind.

Special needs of women cancer patients

Breast cancer can have a profound effect on a woman. Fortunately, new treatments and surgical procedures for breast cancer frequently mean the breast can be saved.

A woman who's had a mastectomy will need to know many practical matters. If her lymph glands have been removed, the arm on that side will always have a decreased ability to fight infection, and she'll have to learn how to take precautions against cuts, sunburns, and similar problems to prevent getting an infection. She'll also have to learn how to do special exercises to reduce swelling and regain muscle tone and the full use of her arm. To improve appearance, a woman may use a prosthetic device, which can do a great deal to restore her self-esteem. She'll need to choose one carefully and have it fitted properly. For some women, breast reconstruction is a possibility: new surgical techniques have made it possible for doctors to virtually rebuild a breast. This can make an immeasurable difference in a woman's feelings about herself and those around her.

Strengthening exercises

After a mastectomy, it's important that you exercise the involved arm and shoulder to prevent muscle shortening, maintain muscle tone, and improve blood and lymph circulation.

Wall climbing

Stand facing a wall, with your toes as close to the wall as possible and your feet apart. Bending your elbows slightly, place your palms against the wall at shoulder level. Then, flexing your fingers, work your hands up the wall until your arms are fully extended. Work your hands back down to the starting point.

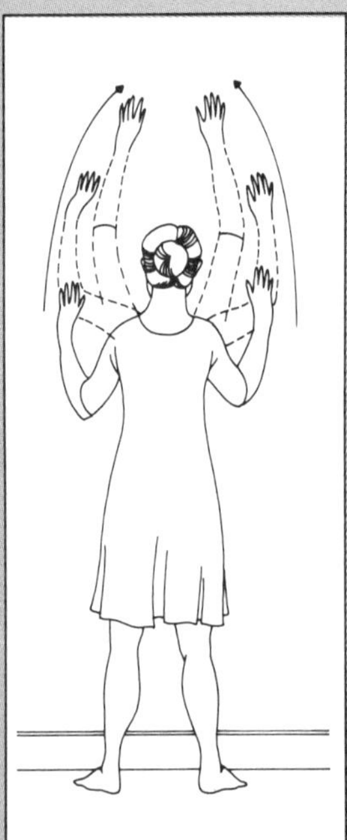

Pendulum swing

Place your uninvolved arm on the back of a chair. Let your involved (free) arm hang loosely.

1. *Swing your arm from left to right. Be sure the movement comes from your shoulder joint and not your elbow.*

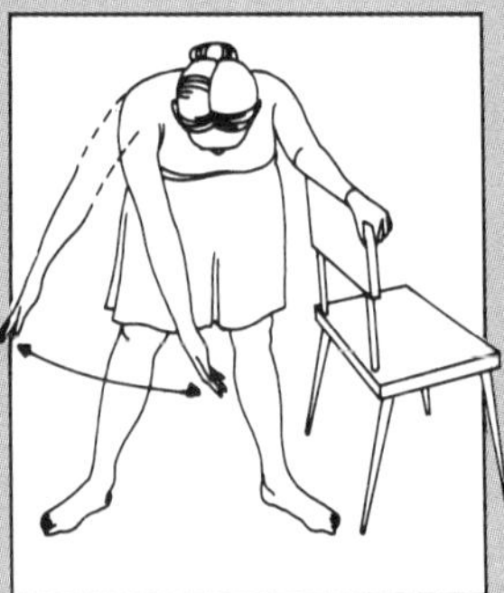

2. *Swing your arm in small circles. Again, be sure the movement is coming from your shoulder joint. As your arm relaxes, the size of the circle will probably increase. Then, circle in the opposite direction.*

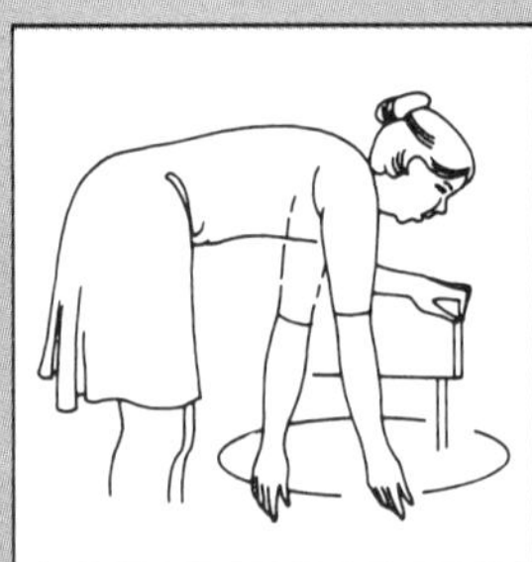

3. *Swing your arm forward and backward from your shoulder, within the range of comfort.*

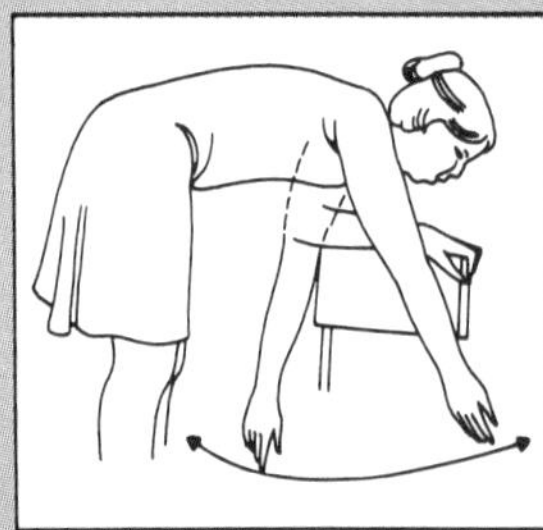

Pully

Toss a rope over your shower curtain rod and hold an end of the rope in each hand. Using a seesaw motion and with your arms outstretched, slide the rope up and down over the rod.

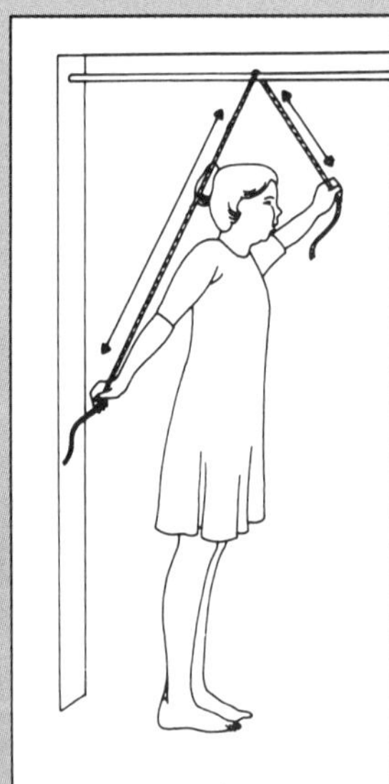

Rope turning
Stand facing the door. Take the free end of a rope in the hand of the operated side. Place your other hand on your hip. With your arm extended and held away from your body, turn the rope, making as wide a swing as possible. Start slowly, and increase your speed as your arm gets stronger.

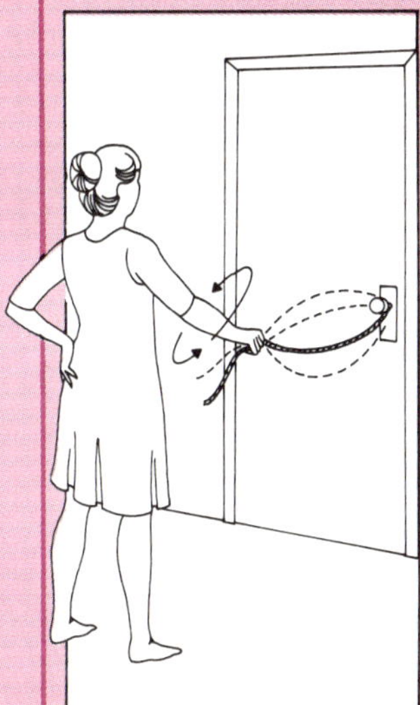

After cancer surgery, a patient will benefit from talking to other patients who've gone through a similar trauma. In one case, a woman went into a deep depression following her mastectomy and resisted all efforts to lift her out of it. Finally, a hospital nurse contacted a local volunteer from the American Cancer Society, who had had both breasts removed. The nurse tracked down the volunteer on a tennis court and convinced her to visit the patient immediately after her game. When the patient saw this cheerful, attractive woman bounce in after a rousing game of tennis, she brightened immediately.

Special needs of ostomy patients

Ostomies are relatively common operations. While these procedures can be very upsetting initially, thousands of ostomy patients live normal lives and are cancer-free. Here again, the patient will benefit from talks with others who've been through the same experience. Ostomy clubs around the country have group meetings and volunteers just for that purpose.

These patients need intensive, sometimes continuous counseling, especially when they're first adjusting to their condition. The spouse should also participate in the counseling, since many people are disturbed by the ostomy when they first see it on someone else. Patients should learn as much as they can before their operation, including care for the wound.

Special needs of children with cancer

Caring for a child with cancer is probably the most devastating experience a parent or a family will have to endure. These children need almost constant parental presence, especially during treatment sessions or if the child is younger than age 5 and can't grasp the concept of serious illness. On the other hand, they need to be treated as normally as possible once they're home. They should return to school, social activities, and chores as soon as they can, so they can feel like normal members of the family once again. Like all cancer patients, children should have their questions answered to the fullest extent of their understanding. The best care and communication will probably come from professionals who specialize in the treatment of childhood cancer.

Teenagers can grasp the seriousness of their disease, but along with it they'll need to deal with issues of interrupted maturation and development of independence, a separate identity, and relationships with the opposite

Understanding colostomy

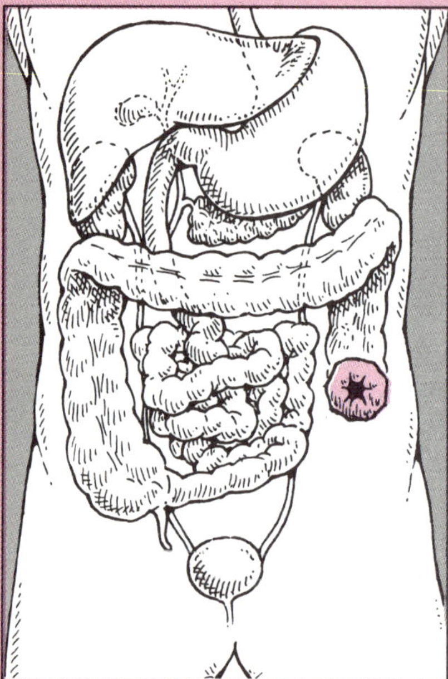

Colostomy

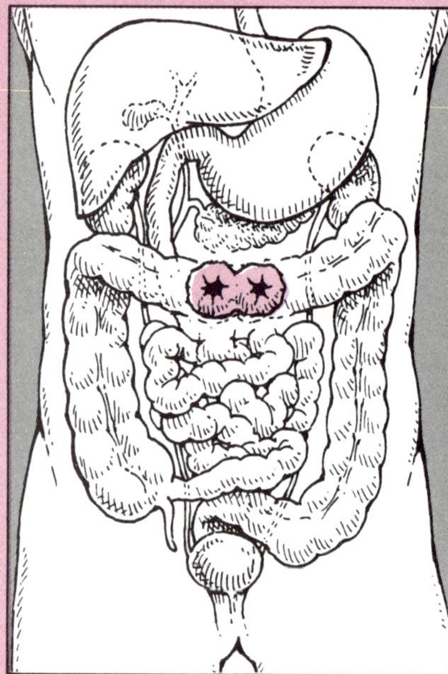

Double colostomy

A colostomy, a kind of ostomy, allows excretion of body wastes through a surgically created opening between the colon and the surface of the body. The surgeon ends the intestine outside the abdomen, creating a stoma, or opening. Wastes collect in the attached ostomy bag. While this procedure may sound extreme, thousands of patients have adjusted to it and within two to three months have resumed swimming, playing tennis, eating a normal diet, and having sexual relations.

A double colostomy is usually temporary, often to let the intestines rest and heal. Later, follow-up surgery reattaches the intestines.

sex. They also must cope with any changes in physical appearance, at a stage in life when appearance is paramount. Many doctors recommend buying wigs before a patient's hair begins to fall out from treatment, so the best color match can be obtained. Very often patients don't need the wig after all, but find support in knowing it's there.

Above all, young cancer patients need to have their fears acknowledged and morale boosted. Family members or professional counselors should encourage them to express their feelings of rage over being so sick, as well as guilt feelings over being a burden to the family. They must be assured that their parents and other family members are behind them, no matter what.

Special needs of terminal cancer patients

Terminally ill patients should be told the truth—if they indicate that's what they want. No matter what the extent of their desire to know, patients should never be lied to, and they should never be given false hope. Many patients can figure out the truth on their own, even if they don't ask about it. They'll know when they're being lied to, and this will only make them suspicious and resentful.

Different people react to the knowledge that they're dying in different ways. Some people withdraw and become depressed, while others resolve to make the most of their remaining time and live each day to the fullest. Elderly patients often accept and discuss the prospect of death more easily than younger patients, who may feel angry or cheated. More than anything else, dying patients are still alive and need to be treated that way. They need loved ones around to remind them that they're still valuable members of society.

Many terminally ill patients elect to spend their final days or weeks in a hospice. A hospice is a facility that specializes in the 24-hour-a-day care of dying people. It may be independently run or located in a nursing home or a hospital. The hospice staff is trained to offer care and support to patients and their families. To patients they offer symptomatic treatment and emotional support; they don't try to cure them or prolong their lives, but rather to make the time they have comfortable and meaningful. After a patient dies, hospice staff members may make home visits to the patient's family for up to two years.

Rehabilitation

The goal of rehabilitation is to return the patient to a normal life. Many programs and organizations offer rehabilitation services, but the patient's attitude ultimately determines how successful the rehabilitation will be. For example, women who have had radical mastectomies should start doing simple tasks like combing their hair no later than 2 weeks after surgery. If they wait any longer, they may not regain a full range of motion in the arm. Similarly, laryngectomy patients should start learning new speech methods before they leave the hospital.

In short, patients need to make as much use as possible of the rehabilitation services available to them. This will hasten their resumption of regular activities and help them to feel normal once again.

When someone you love has cancer

Family members of cancer patients have needs that, if not met, can take a severe emotional toll. A patient's family has the right to know all they can about his or her disease. Ideally, they should be given the same information the patient receives. Armed with this information, they must adjust to at least temporary changes in family roles. For example, the loss of the family nurturer or breadwinner means that others will have to assume more responsibility.

Each family member reacts to this crisis in his or her own way. Almost everyone will feel some combination of shock, fear, denial, guilt, and anxiety, but different people express these feelings in different ways and in different intensities. Relatives who thought they knew one another intimately may be surprised at the

What is a hospice?

The hospice philosophy is simple: to maintain the dignity of the dying patient and the patient's family through the patient's death, as well as to help family members through their period of bereavement. The hospice aims to improve patient and family comfort and well-being until death occurs, instead of prolonging life for its own sake.

A hospice typically employs a multidisciplinary team, including doctors, nurses, volunteers, clergy, a nutritionist, a homemaker/home-health aide, social workers, and other professionals as needed. At the core of the team is the patient and his or her family.

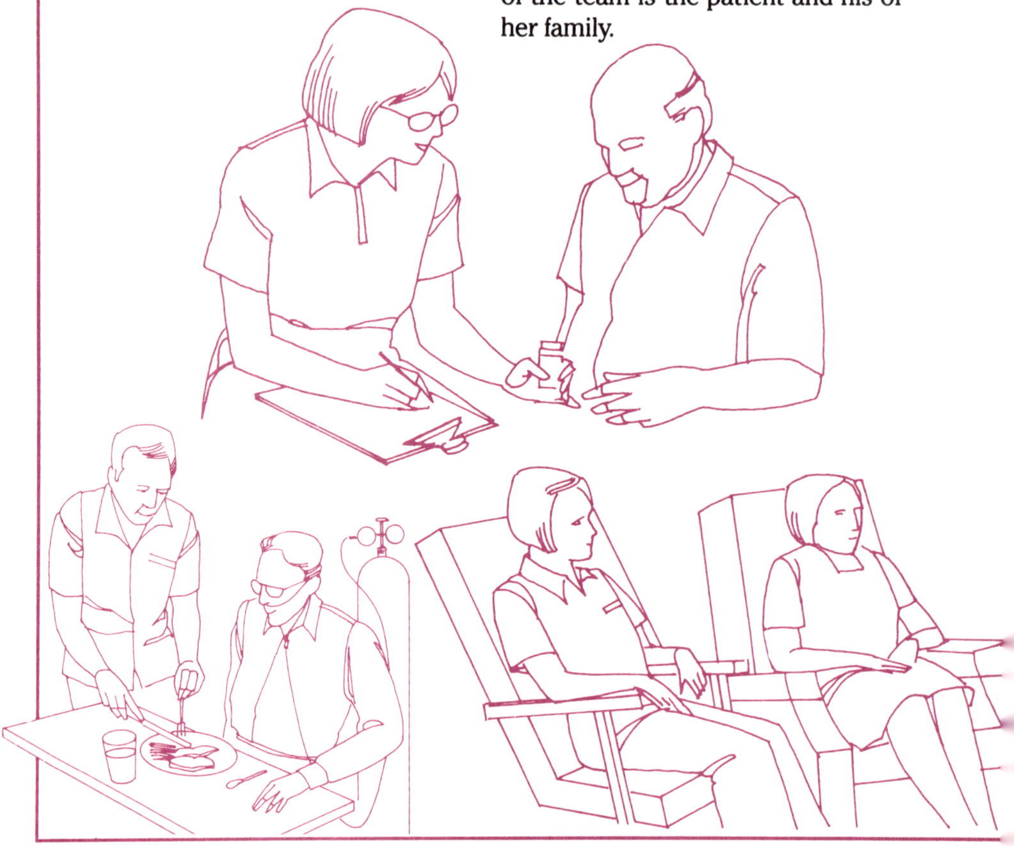

changes in behavior that occur when a cancer crisis takes place. Different people have different coping styles that must be tolerated and respected. While a cancer patient is hospitalized, the family usually adjusts to the absence. When the patient returns home, they have to readjust all over. Often they must learn how to perform new tasks, like preparing special meals or changing wound dressings. A patient's loved ones have to strike the balance between helping the person stay as independent as possible while not ap-

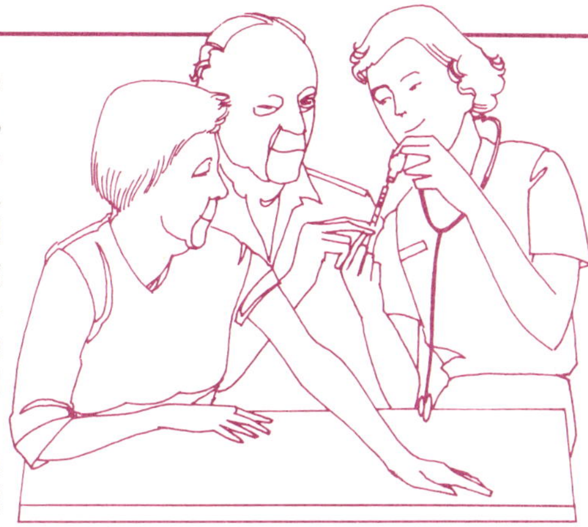

Team members are available around the clock, seven days a week, to care for the patient and the patient's family as an inseparable unit. They administer to the patient's and family's physical needs—controlling distress from the signs and symptoms of the disease, especially the pain—and they address emotional and spiritual needs.

Although a hospice may exist in a separate institution or special unit of a hospital, the ideal setting is usually the patient's home. Regardless of size or location, all hospices try to maintain as close to a normal life-style as possible in a homelike setting.

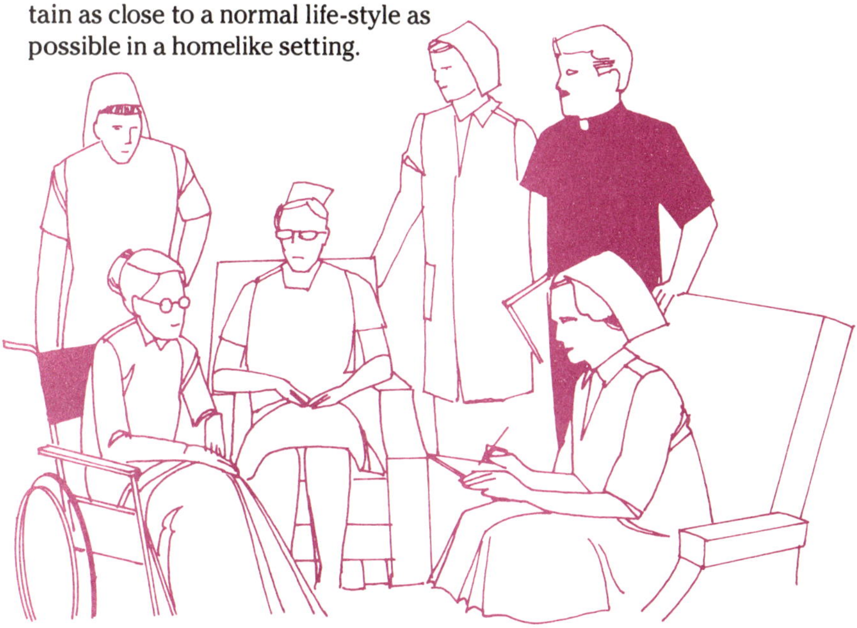

pearing insensitive to emotional needs. Some anger and resentment are inevitable and normal. Professional counselors encourage relatives to express these feelings while trying to minimize guilt.

A family's readjustment may be even more difficult if the patient's appearance is changed in some way, as often occurs after surgery for cancer of the head or neck. Here again, feelings of repugnance are normal but lead to a lot of guilt. Loved ones may also feel guilt if they start worrying about their own needs, like the potential loss of emotional and financial support, as well as a need for a break from the demanding daily routine. In all of these cases, the best help is to discuss these fears and feelings with a close friend, a religious adviser, or a counselor.

Children of a cancer patient should be told the truth about their parent's disease. This is true even for very young children, who may secretly feel they were in some way responsible for what's wrong with Mommy or Daddy. Support groups now exist for children of cancer patients. They answer questions and help youngsters cope with the disruption of normal life. These groups provide counseling and group support for children as young as age 3.

For the parents of a child with cancer, some professional counseling is almost always advisable. Each parent undergoes very different forms of stress: the experience could destroy the marriage. If the child dies, each parent may grieve in a way that may be misinterpreted or resented by the other. This could be a time that draws a couple closer together, but it may also pull them apart. This can be avoided if the parents find someone they can talk to and if they make a real effort at communication throughout the illness.

The hospice

The first modern-day hospice was started at St. Luke's Hospital in England. In the United States today are nearly 200 hospice programs. Not all of these are located in outside institutions: many provide care in the patient's own home. Regardless of where the hospice service is located, it differs from an ordinary medical care facility in several ways. The hospice provides a homey atmosphere: unlimited visits are allowed, even from pets. If located outside the home, hospices are usually equipped with living rooms and kitchens. Many dying patients are happiest in hospices because they receive around-the-clock care, they're with others who share their plight, and they feel less like burdens to family and friends.

Returning to normal life

Each year, more and more cancer patients leave the hospital as cured, fully functioning individuals, eager and able to get on with the business of living. Returning to everyday life may require physical, emotional, and vocational rehabilitation, but it can be done. The ease of a patient's readjustment seems to depend most on the strength of the family ties and the depth of individual religious or philosophical beliefs. Age, education, socioeconomic status, and change in appearance can't be used to predict how easy or difficult a patient's readjustment will be.

When returning to work, cancer patients may have to deal with some prejudice from coworkers, who may think the patient needs special help or a lighter work load. According to some studies, however, cancer victims often work harder, perhaps as a way of proving themselves. Every time a cured cancer patient returns to society, he or she helps chip away at the block of fear that most people have erected against cancer. And as doctors learn more about cancer prevention, treatment, and rehabilitation, more and more of these people will be around.

Guilt

Guilt is difficult to deal with. It can come from a thousand different sources. What makes it so difficult in all cases, though, is that so often you can't take any specific action to absolve it. Only time seems to truly resolve the feeling.

For more information

The American Cancer Society
National Headquarters: 777 Third Avenue
New York, NY 10017
(212) 586-8700
The ACS is a voluntary organization dedicated to the control and eradication of cancer. The society runs an extensive public education program and provides many free pamphlets and publications. It offers these rehabilitation services:

- The International Association of Laryngectomies
- Reach to Recovery (for mastectomy patients)
- The Ostomy Rehabilitation Program

The National Cancer Institute
Toll-free hot line: 1-800-4-CANCER
The NCI is the branch of the National Institutes of Health charged with cancer research and public cancer education. You can use its 24-hour hot line for free information, including details about children's hospitals around the country.

Free booklets on helping children to understand cancer

"Helping Children Understand," a guide for parents
American Cancer Society, Minnesota Division
3316 West 66th Street
Minneapolis, MN 55435

"Helping Children Cope When Parents Have Cancer"
American Cancer Society, Massachusetts Division
247 Commonwealth Avenue
Boston, MA 02116

"When Someone in Your Family Has Cancer"
National Cancer Institute
Building 31, Room 10A18
Bethesda, MD 20205

Local resources

Your doctor or the public affairs office of your hospital can guide you to local psychologists, volunteers, and support groups.

Index